Rapid Response Systems & Fluid Resuscitation

Editors

MICHAEL A. DeVITA
ANDREW D. SHAW
SEAN M. BAGSHAW

CRITICAL CARE CLINICS

www.criticalcare.theclinics.com

Consulting Editor
JOHN A. KELLUM

April 2018 • Volume 34 • Number 2

ELSEVIER

1600 John F. Kennedy Boulevard • Suite 1800 • Philadelphia, Pennsylvania, 19103-2899

http://www.theclinics.com

CRITICAL CARE CLINICS Volume 34, Number 2
April 2018 ISSN 0749-0704, ISBN-13: 978-0-323-58300-8

Editor: Colleen Dietzler
Developmental Editor: Casey Potter

Critical Care Clinics (ISSN: 0749-0704) is published quarterly by Elsevier Inc., 360 Park Avenue South, New York, NY 10010-1710. Months of issue are January, April, July, and October. Business and Editorial Offices: 1600 John F. Kennedy Blvd., Suite 1800, Philadelphia, PA 19103-2899. Customer Service Office: 6277 Sea Harbor Drive, Orlando, FL 32887-4800. Periodicals postage paid at New York, NY and additional mailing offices. Subscription prices are $234.00 per year for US individuals, $619.00 per year for US institution, $100.00 per year for US students and residents, $279.00 per year for Canadian individuals, $776.00 per year for Canadian institutions, $309.00 per year for international individuals, $776.00 per year for international institutions and $150.00 per year for Canadian and foreign students/residents. To receive student/resident rate, orders must be accompanied by name of affiliated institution, date of term, and the signature of program/residency coordinator on institution letterhead. Orders will be billed at individual rate until proof of status is received. Foreign air speed delivery is included in all *Clinics* subscription prices. All prices are subject to change without notice. POSTMASTER: Send address changes to *Critical Care Clinics*, Elsevier Periodicals Customer Service, 11830 Westline Industrial Drive, St. Louis, MO 63146. **Customer Service: 1-800-654-2452 (US). From outside of the US, call 1-314-447-8871. Fax: 1-314-447-8029. E-mail: journalscustomerservice-usa@ elsevier.com (for print support) or journalsonlinesupport-usa@elsevier.com (for online support).**

Reprints. For copies of 100 or more of articles in this publication, please contact the Commercial Reprints Department, Elsevier Inc., 360 Park Avenue South, New York, NY 10010-1710. Tel.: 212-633-3874; Fax: 212-633-3820; E-mail: reprints@elsevier.com.

Critical Care Clinics is also published in Spanish by Editorial Inter-Medica, Junin 917, 1er A, 1113, Buenos Aires, Argentina.

Critical Care Clinics is covered in *MEDLINE/PubMed (Index Medicus), EMBASE/Excerpta Medica, Current Concepts/Clinical Medicine, ISI/BIOMED,* and *Chemical Abstracts.*

Contributors

CONSULTING EDITOR

JOHN A. KELLUM, MD, MCCM
Professor of Critical Care Medicine, Medicine, Bioengineering and Clinical & Translational Science, Director, Center for Critical Care Nephrology, Vice Chair for Research, Department of Critical Care Medicine, University of Pittsburgh School of Medicine, Pittsburgh, Pennsylvania, USA

EDITORS

MICHAEL A. DeVITA, MD, FCCM, FRCP, FACP
Director, Critical Care, Harlem Hospital Center, New York, New York, USA

ANDREW D. SHAW, MB, FRCA, FFICM, FCCM, MMHC
Chair, Department of Anesthesiology and Pain Medicine, Faculty of Medicine and Dentistry, University of Alberta, Edmonton, Alberta, Canada

SEAN M. BAGSHAW, MD, MSc, FRCPC
Chair (Interim), Department of Critical Care Medicine, Faculty of Medicine and Dentistry, University of Alberta, Edmonton, Alberta, Canada

AUTHORS

MUSTAFA AL-MASHAT, MD
Critical Care Fellow, Department of Internal Medicine, The George Washington University, Washington, DC, USA

SABRINA ARSHED, MD
Postdoctoral Fellow, Department of Critical Care Medicine, University of Pittsburgh, Pittsburgh, Pennsylvania, USA

RINALDO BELLOMO, MBBS (Hons), MD, FRACP, FCICM, FAAHMS
Director of Research, Department of Intensive Care, Austin Hospital, Professor and Co-Director, Australian and New Zealand Intensive Care Research Centre, Department of Epidemiology and Preventive Medicine, Monash University, Professor, Doctor of Medicine, The University of Melbourne, Melbourne, Victoria, Australia

ALEXANDRA BRIGGS, MD
Acute Care Surgery Fellow, Department of Surgery, University of Pittsburgh, Pittsburgh, Pennsylvania, USA

RENEE COVER, BSN, RN, CPHRM
Risk Manager, Johns Hopkins Health System Legal Department, The Johns Hopkins Hospital, Baltimore, Maryland, USA

PATRICIA L. DALBY, MD
Associate Professor, Department of Anesthesiology, University of Pittsburgh School of Medicine, Magee-Womens Hospital of UPMC, Pittsburgh, Pennsylvania, USA

MICHAEL A. DeVITA, MD, FCCM, FRCP, FACP
Director, Critical Care, Harlem Hospital Center, New York, New York, USA

JORDAN DUVAL-ARNOULD, MPH, DrPH
The Johns Hopkins University School of Medicine, Johns Hopkins Medicine Simulation Center, Baltimore, Maryland, USA

NEIL J. GLASSFORD, BScMedSci (Hons), MBChB, PhD, MRCP(UK), AAAHMS
Registrar and Research Fellow, Department of Intensive Care, Austin Hospital, Adjunct Senior Research Fellow, Department of Epidemiology and Preventive Medicine, Monash University, Australian and New Zealand Intensive Care Research Centre, Melbourne, Victoria, Australia

GABRIELLA GOSMAN, MD
Associate Professor, Department of Obstetrics and Gynecology, University of Pittsburgh School of Medicine, Magee-Womens Hospital of UPMC, Pittsburgh, Pennsylvania, USA

KURT HERZER, MD, PhD
Physician Scientist, Oscar Health, Brooklyn, New York, USA

KENNETH HILLMAN, AO, MBBS, MD, FRCA, FCICM, FRCP
Professor of Intensive Care, Liverpool Hospital, South Western Sydney Clinical School, Director, Simpson Centre for Health Services Research, University of New South Wales, Ingham Institute for Applied Medical Research, Liverpool, New South Wales, Australia

LARS BROKSØ HOLST, MD, PhD
Department of Intensive Care, Copenhagen University Hospital, Rigshospitalet, Copenhagen Ø, Denmark

TAMMY JU, MD
Resident Physician, Department of Surgery, The George Washington University, Washington, DC, USA

LAEBEN LESTER, MD
Assistant Professor, Departments of Anesthesiology and Critical Care Medicine and Emergency Medicine, Associate Medical Director, Johns Hopkins Medicine Multidisciplinary Airway Programs, Johns Hopkins Medicine, Baltimore, Maryland, USA

LYNETTE MARK, MD
Associate Professor, Department of Anesthesiology and Critical Care Medicine, Joint Appointment, Department of Otolaryngology–Head and Neck Surgery, Executive Medical Director, Johns Hopkins Medicine Multidisciplinary Airway Programs, Director, Difficult Airway Response Team (DART) Program, Johns Hopkins Medicine, Baltimore, Maryland, USA

HEATHER NEWTON, BS, RN
Clinical Data Abstractor, Resuscitation Events, The Johns Hopkins Hospital, Baltimore, Maryland, USA

ANDREW B. PEITZMAN, MD
Distinguished Professor of Surgery, Mark M. Ravitch Professor and Vice Chairman, Department of Surgery, UPMC Vice President for Trauma and Surgical Services, University of Pittsburgh School of Medicine, Pittsburgh, Pennsylvania, USA

ANDERS PERNER, MD, PhD
Department of Intensive Care, Copenhagen University Hospital, Rigshospitalet, Copenhagen Ø, Denmark; Centre for Research in Intensive Care (CRIC), Denmark

MICHAEL R. PINSKY, MD, CM, Dr hc
Professor, Department of Critical Care Medicine, University of Pittsburgh, Pittsburgh, Pennsylvania, USA

LISBI RIVAS, MD
Resident Physician, Department of Surgery, The George Washington University, Washington, DC, USA

MARK ROMIG, MD
Johns Hopkins University School of Medicine, Johns Hopkins Medicine, Armstrong Institute for Patient Safety and Quality, Baltimore, Maryland, USA

SOFIE LOUISE RYGÅRD, MD
Department of Intensive Care, Copenhagen University Hospital, Rigshospitalet, Copenhagen Ø, Denmark

ADAM SAPIRSTEIN, MD
Johns Hopkins University School of Medicine, Johns Hopkins Medicine, Armstrong Institute for Patient Safety and Quality, Baltimore, Maryland, USA

BABAK SARANI, MD, FACS, FCCM
Director of the Center for Trauma and Critical Care, Associate Professor, Department of Surgery, The George Washington University, Washington, DC, USA

BRIAN C. SPENCE, MD, MHCDS
Associate Professor, Department of Anesthesiology, Dartmouth Geisel School of Medicine, Dartmouth-Hitchcock Medical Center, Lebanon, New Hampshire, USA

ANDREAS H. TAENZER, MS, MD
Associate Professor of Anesthesiology and Pediatrics, The Dartmouth Institute, Dartmouth Geisel School of Medicine, The Dartmouth Institute for Health Policy & Clinical Practice, Dartmouth-Hitchcock Medical Center, Lebanon, New Hampshire, USA

BRADFORD D. WINTERS, PhD, MD
Johns Hopkins University School of Medicine, Johns Hopkins Medicine, Armstrong Institute for Patient Safety and Quality, Baltimore, Maryland, USA

KIM MOI WONG LAMA, MD
Assistant Professor, Department of Internal Medicine, Columbia University College of Physicians and Surgeons, Harlem Hospital Center, New York, New York, USA

Contents

Section I: Rapid Response Systems
Edited By: Michael A. DeVita

> The prevention of adverse events continues to be the focus of patient
> safety work. Although rapid response systems have improved the efferent
> limb of the patient's rescue, the detection of the patient's deterioration (the
> afferent limb) has not been solved. This article provides an overview of the
> complex issues surrounding patient surveillance by addressing the prin-
> cipal considerations of continuous monitoring as they relate to implemen-
> tation, choice of sensors and physiologic variables, notification, and alarm
> balancing, as well as future research opportunities.

> Electronic medical records can be used to mine clinical data (big data),
> providing automated analysis during patient care. This article describes
> the source and potential impact of big data analysis on risk stratification
> and early detection of deterioration. It compares use of big data analysis
> with existing methods of identifying at-risk patients who require rapid
> response. Aggregate weighted scoring systems combined with big data
> analysis offer an opportunity to detect clinical changes that precede rapid
> response team activation. Future studies must determine if this will
> decrease transfers to intensive care units and cardiac arrests on the floors.

> *Failure to rescue* is death occurring after a complication. Rapid response
> teams developed as a prompt intervention for patients with early clinical
> deterioration, generally from medical conditions or complications. Patients
> with surgical complications or surgical pathology require prompt evalua-
> tion and management by surgeons to avoid deterioration; this is *surgical
> rescue*. Patients in the medical intensive care unit may develop intraabdo-
> minal pathology that requires expeditious operative intervention. Acute
> care surgeons should serve as the surgical rapid response team to help
> assess and manage these complex patients. Collaboration between

intensivists and surgeons is essential to rescue patients from complications and surgical disease.

Patricia L. Dalby and Gabriella Gosman

An obstetric-specific crisis team allows institutions to optimize the care response for patients with emergent maternal or fetal needs. Characteristics of optimal obstetric rapid response teams are team member role designations; streamlined communication; prompt access to resources; ongoing education, rehearsal, and training; and continual team quality analysis. The outcomes must be incorporated into team responses and reinforced in training. Team response provides a key resource to reassure staff, physicians, and patients that prompt crisis care is only a single call away. Data show that team activation is common, improves the care process, and has promise to improve outcomes.

Lynette Mark, Laeben Lester, Renee Cover, and Kurt Herzer

A decade ago the Difficult Airway Response Team (DART) program was created at the Johns Hopkins Hospital as a multidisciplinary effort to address airway-related adverse events in the nonoperative setting. Root cause analysis of prior events indicated that a major factor in adverse patient outcomes was lack of a systematic approach for responding to difficult airway patients in an emergency. The DART program encompasses operational, safety, and educational initiatives and has responded to approximately 1000 events since its initiation, with no resultant adult airway-related adverse events or morbidity. This article provides lessons learned and recommendations for initiating a DART program.

Tammy Ju, Mustafa Al-Mashat, Lisbi Rivas, and Babak Sarani

Sepsis rapid response teams are being incorporated into hospitals around the world. Based on the concept of the medical emergency team, the sepsis rapid response team consists of a specifically trained team of health care providers educated in the early recognition, diagnosis, and treatment of patients at risk of having or who have sepsis. Using hospital-wide initiatives consisting of multidisciplinary education, training, and specific resource utilization, such teams have been found to improve patient outcomes.

Mark Romig, Jordan Duval-Arnould, Bradford D. Winters, Heather Newton, and Adam Sapirstein

To better support the highest function of the Johns Hopkins Hospital adult code and rapid response teams, a team leadership role was created for a faculty intensivist, with the intention to integrate and improve processes of care delivery, documentation, and decision making. This article examines process and outcomes associated with the introduction of this role. It demonstrates that an intensivist has the potential to improve patient care while offsetting costs through improved billing capture.

Section II: Fluid Resuscitation

Edited By: Andrew D. Shaw and Sean M. Bagshaw

Fluids during resuscitation from shock increase the mean systemic pressure and venous return. The pressure gradient for venous return must increase. Mean systemic pressure is the amount of vascular space in unstressed and stressed volume, mostly unstressed. Shock states can decrease the mean systemic pressure by increasing the unstressed volume, decreasing the total blood volume, or decreasing the pressure gradient for venous return. Crystalloids across bodily spaces restore normal volume, whereas colloids remain in the intravascular space. The electrolyte content of fluids matters, and excess chloride impairs renal blood flow. Albumin seems to be more effective at restoring blood volume in severe sepsis but not in other conditions.

Acute kidney injury (AKI) is common, although commonly used clinical diagnostic markers are imperfect. Intravenous fluid administration remains a cornerstone of therapy worldwide, but there is minimal evidence of efficacy for the use of fluid bolus therapy outside of specific circumstances, and emerging evidence associates fluid accumulation with worse renal outcomes and even increased mortality among critically ill patients. Artificial colloid solutions have been associated with harm, and chloride-rich solutions may adversely affect renal function. Large trials to provide guidance regarding the optimal fluid choices to prevent or ameliorate AKI, and promote renal recovery, are urgently required.

The critical care and perioperative settings are high consumers of blood products, with multiple units and different products often given to an individual patient. The recommendation of this article is always to consider the risks and benefits for a specific blood product for a specific patient in a specific clinical setting. Optimize patient status by treating anemia and preventing the need for red blood cell transfusion. Consider other options for correction of anemia and coagulation disorders, and use an imperative non-overtransfusion policy for all blood products.

Rapid Response Systems & Fluid Resuscitation

CRITICAL CARE CLINICS

Section I: Rapid Response Systems
Edited By: Michael A. DeVita

Preface

Why RRS? Where RRS?

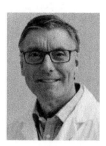

Michael A. DeVita, MD, FCCM, FRCP, FACP
Editor

The concept of rapid response systems (RRSs) was first imagined after a 19-year-old woman bled to death on a general ward of a major teaching hospital. There had been a slow but obvious increase in respiratory and pulse rate, and a decrease in blood pressure. The nurses informed the intern, who informed the resident, who informed the surgeon, who was operating in the operating room. By the time the surgeon saw her, she had arrested. She had slowly exsanguinated. This event resulted in no changes in the process of care. Years later, in Australia, Dr Hillman developed the first RRS, the medical emergency team (MET). It was designed to recognize and respond to deteriorating patients *before* they suffered serious adverse events. It was a "preemptive strike," in essence sending the "code team" before the code.

The RRS is a process that uses standard objective criteria to define the at-risk patient. It cuts across the usual hospital silos and hierarchies and addresses the needs of the patient with a specialized team. The RRS moves the skills and equipment out of the ICU to create an ICU-like environment anywhere. While most ward clinicians are skillful, they are not there all the time, and they may not be trained in critical illness. The earliest RRS implementers had an uphill battle: they showed that the MET was needed, but in doing so implied that the usual system was a problem. There was significant pushback.

Now rapid response teams are commonplace and often required by governmental or regulatory bodies. How to organize the team is well reported, and there are a number of textbooks available. The RRS has been shown to have value for the treatment of *many* critical situations, and some hospitals now have a number of different RRTs for a variety of time-critical situations, including "stroke teams," "coronary syndrome teams," and "sepsis teams." They are effective and have saved innumerable lives worldwide.

RRSs share four cornerstones: an ability to detect critical abnormality and trigger a response, a response of equipment and personnel, an analysis of events to help

Crit Care Clin 34 (2018) xi–xii
https://doi.org/10.1016/j.ccc.2018.01.001
0749-0704/18/© 2018 Published by Elsevier Inc.

prevent future events through usual quality improvement mechanisms, and administrative leadership.

In this *Critical Care Clinics*, the articles explore ways that the concept of RRSs has now expanded to operate in different settings. The articles have two foci. The first highlights the state-of-the-art in monitoring and triggering. It is increasingly recognized that without a reliable and sensitive detection system, no RRS can possibly exist, let alone succeed. Dr Wong Lama and colleagues describe efforts to organize the gigantic amount of data that exists in the electronic health record to enable analysis and prediction. The work on "big data" is promising. It is hoped it will be able to diagnose syndromes that might be missed or recognized late, including recognizing very early deterioration to prevent the need to respond emergently. Another approach to early detection, reported herein by Dr Taenzer and colleagues, emphasizes the use of continuous physiologic monitoring to "fill in the gaps" that occur when vital signs are obtained intermittently. The gaps can miss deterioration of some patients, leading to disastrous results. We expect that continuous monitoring will someday be a standard of care for all hospitalized patients.

The second cluster of articles relates to some critical, focused applications of the RRS. The situations share a need for speed, organization, and accuracy of care. Dr Sarani describes sepsis teams; Dr Mark explores the difficult airway response team, and Dr Dalby describes the experience with an obstetric rapid response team. Finally, Drs Briggs and Peitzman discuss surgical rapid response teams. While the authors hope that readers will be able to emulate them at their organization, we also hope that readers will find commonalities in the RRS approach and apply those principles to other situations.

Dr Hillman and I share another desire: nobody should die in hospital unexpectedly. The cardiac-arrest-rate goal should be zero. We recognize that of course some patients in hospital will and must die. For those patients, the deaths should be expected, prepared for, and treated with care and comfort.

Hospital acuity is increasing, and the process of care is increasingly complex. The need for reorganization of hospital care into clusters of goal-directed rapid response teams is becoming more apparent. We may be near the tipping point for this reorganization.

Michael A. DeVita, MD, FCCM, FRCP, FACP
Harlem Hospital Center
506 Lenox Avenue
New York, NY 10037, USA

Kenneth Hillman, AO, MBBS, MD, FRCA, FCICM, FRCP
Simpson Center for Safety
PO Box 3154
Liverpool, NSW 2170, Australia

E-mail addresses:
Michael.devita@nychhc.org (M.A. DeVita)
k.hillman@unsw.edu.au (K. Hillman)

The Afferent Limb of Rapid Response Systems

Continuous Monitoring on General Care Units

Andreas H. Taenzer, MS, MD[a],*, Brian C. Spence, MD, MHCDS[b]

KEYWORDS

- Rapid response systems ● Continuous monitoring ● Alarm management
- Physiologic sensors

KEY POINTS

- Continuous monitoring is the way to solve the afferent limb problem and to improve rapid response systems.
- Implementation, education, and training are key elements in determining the success.
- Sensors are only as good as their tolerance by patients.
- Alarm management is a key consideration for surveillance monitoring.

INTRODUCTION

Patients in general care units (GCUs) often deteriorate unnoticed while under our care, leading to preventable adverse events and escalation of care.[1,2] Many of these adverse events are preceded by changes in vital signs and hence provide opportunity for earlier intervention.[3,4] Rapid response systems (RRSs) were introduced to intervene at an earlier stage than at cardiorespiratory arrest (code teams).[5] **Fig. 1** illustrates the deterioration process and the points of intervention for code and rapid response teams (RRTs), as well as patient surveillance. The success of RRS, however, is dependent on being activated, a process that depends on 2 key components: monitoring and notification, or the "afferent limb."[6]

Although there have been successful implementations of surveillance and continuous monitoring systems on GCUs, to reduce inpatient adverse events, by using pulse oximetry–based surveillance for almost a decade,[7] the understanding of surveillance monitoring and its utilization of principles of population health medicine to hospital

[a] Department of Anesthesiology, The Geisel School of Medicine at Dartmouth, The Dartmouth Institute for Health Policy and Clinical Practice, Dartmouth Hitchcock Medical Center, One Medical Center Drive, Lebanon, NH 03756, USA; [b] Department of Anesthesiology, The Geisel School of Medicine at Dartmouth, Dartmouth Hitchcock Medical Center, One Medical Center Drive, Lebanon, NH 03756, USA
* Corresponding author.
E-mail address: andreas.h.taenzer@dartmouth.edu

Crit Care Clin 34 (2018) 189–198
https://doi.org/10.1016/j.ccc.2017.12.001
0749-0704/18/© 2017 Elsevier Inc. All rights reserved.

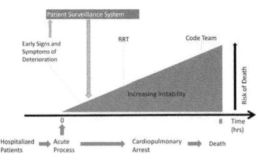

Fig. 1. Illustration of increasing physiologic deterioration over 8 hours, ultimately leading to cardiac arrest and death. Code teams intervene at the time of arrest, RRTs intervene earlier during the process and patient surveillance was introduced to halt the deterioration at an even earlier time point while being integrated in the workflow with RRTs. (*From* Taenzer AH, Pyke JB, McGrath SP. A review of current and emerging approaches to address failure-to-rescue. Anesthesiology 2011;115:421–31; with permission.)

wards is still in its infancy. The practice of risk stratifying individual patients based on comorbidities has largely failed because the risk environment that a patient is being exposed to is much more complex than just the patient's comorbidities on which the stratifications are primarily based.[1,8]

Postoperative patients on opioids are a subset of the inpatient population at particularly high risk for preventable adverse events due to respiratory depression.[9] Postoperative respiratory failure represents nearly 11% of all inpatient safety events and has the highest mortality rate per 100 discharges of all classified safety events.[10,11] According to the Joint Commission's Sentinel Event database (2004–2011), 47% of respiratory depression events were wrong dosing medication errors, 29% were related to improper monitoring of the patient, and 11% were related to other factors, including excessive dosing, medication interactions, and adverse drug reactions (http://www.jointcommission.org/sentinel_event_statistics/, last accessed April 9, 2017). These data provide some insight as to why risk stratification and selective, individual monitoring has failed, as individual risk profiles do not accurately account for the entire risk environment. In the example of postoperative respiratory depression, almost half of events are related to medication administration (not ordering) error. Based on these considerations with respect to patient surveillance, the continuous monitoring of all patients (vs a selected group based on individual risk stratification) was introduced a decade ago.[1,7,8]

CONTINUOUS MONITORING

Intermittent sampling of vital signs, the current practice, is insufficient to detect physiologic deterioration processes in a timely fashion to prompt interventions. This is often cited as the primary reason for "unexpected" adverse events in patients.[12] Episodic vital sign collection, even when sampled in 2-hour intervals, has been shown to miss adverse events in postsurgical patients.[13] Additionally, most manually collected vital signs are inaccurate and fail to reflect the patient's true physiologic state.[14–18] **Fig. 2** illustrates an example of patients on GCUs whose oxygen saturation averaged less than 90% for at least 15 minutes, along with a spot check of oxygen saturation during the same time.[15] Although a systematic review of continuous versus intermittent vital signs monitoring has failed to demonstrate benefits of continuous

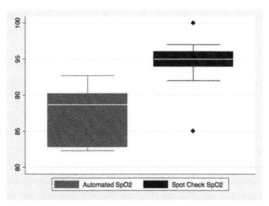

Fig. 2. Box plot demonstrating the distribution of automated versus spot check oxygen saturation sampling of general care unit patients with oxygen saturation averaging less than 90% for more than 15 minutes. Boxes cover first to third quartiles, with median marked by the central line. Whiskers extend to cover 5% to 95% of data, with outliers marked by circles.

monitoring,[19] the evaluation of research studies is severely limited by the focus on published outcomes without appropriate insight into education, workflow integration, and alarm management of surveillance systems. These integral components of deploying complex continuous monitoring systems find little interest in quantitative journals, yet are essential in assessing why continuous monitoring has or has not succeeded. Frontline care providers who are responsible for attaching patients to monitoring systems are nurses, who may have to convince patients of the benefits of continuous monitoring. Unless they perceive this to be advantageous for their patients, as well as their own nursing tasks, they will be reluctant to do so. Health care providers are saturated with competing priorities, and to engage in additional projects, clear benefits must be identified. In task-rich environments, processes that are perceived to be cumbersome and inefficient are likely to fail. Stakeholders need to be engaged in the design of the system to ensure success and sustainability. Basic system engineering standards of creating feedback loops must be taken into account and used as well.

Ideally, baseline data should be captured and stored. In the setting of surveillance systems, this is the normal distribution of vital signs in a population,[20] along with trigger values and characteristics of the measured variable that will indicate when an alert or intervention is required. This information must then be relayed to the monitoring individual, not in the form of raw data, but in a simple instruction set that is both meaningful to the recipient with regard to the message, as well as the importance to attend to the problem (eg, "low heart rate bed 54"). The next step in the feedback relies on the assessment skills of the nurses. They are alerted to a patient's bedside and need to assess and take action. This may be an intervention, such as calling the rapid response team, repositioning the patient, administering medication, or a nonaction. Ideally, alerts and alarms, as well as missed opportunities, are reviewed along with suboptimal and successful interventions on a regular basis to provide feedback to the system stakeholders and generate educational content for the users.

Continuous monitoring in GCUs is likely to gain interest as admitted patients are older and medically more complex than in the past.[21] These patients are more likely to deteriorate and require escalation of care.[22] As pressures on health care systems increase with this higher patient acuity, patient surveillance is needed in low-resourced personnel areas, such as GCUs, to prevent adverse events.[23]

Desirable Properties of Sensors and the Continuous Monitoring System

As these systems are intended to be used around the clock by patients and personnel, certain properties of sensors and system are desirable. Ideally, the sensor is comfortable and hardly noticeable when worn by the patient, is untethered, has long intervals between battery charges, accurately and precisely measures the physiologic variable without artifacts, and transmits the data while preserving full data integrity to a location for further processing. Integration with the electronic medical record would reduce the burden on nursing staff and increase the accuracy of manually entering vital signs.[15,24] The ideal system also would allow the customization of alarm triggers and delays of individual parameters, as well as of the overall system to optimize the alarm performance.[25]

Basic functionality and individualized alarm settings using learning algorithms based on artificial intelligence (AI) is currently a more advanced state **(Fig. 3)**. Under this system, adverse event performance would be optimized per patient based on previous learnings for a large patient population with no user input (AI). Continuously sampled vital sign data would be integrated with comorbidities, laboratory results, medications, and interpretation of text mining of nursing and physician notes. All of these data would be readily available for educational feedback and quality control for clinicians, as well as being displayed on a clinically meaningful dashboard for review.

Physiologic Variables in Continuous Monitoring

When considering various physiologic variables to monitor, the availability of sensors with the properties discussed previously must be considered. Monitoring of tidal volumes, for example, may be desirable, but no adequate sensor in nonintubated patients is available. Exhaled carbon dioxide may serve as a proxy for minute ventilation, but it poorly reflects end-tidal CO_2,[9] and nasal cannulas are poorly tolerated by patients.[8] Much of the basic research that allows insight into the normal distribution of vital signs in an inpatient population has not been completed until recently with the ability to store and analyze large amounts of data.[26] This newly available data has not been sufficiently linked to adverse events to identify which vital signs should be monitored as of yet.[1] New technology, such as sound-based respiratory rate monitoring, can meet many of the previously described requirements for accuracy, patient tolerance, and minimizing artifacts, but may nevertheless provide only limited value over other physiologic variables already monitored, as we found when adding respiratory rate to an already existing pulse oximetry–based surveillance system.[27]

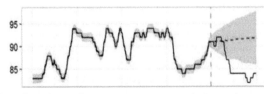

Fig. 3. Using machine learning to forecast oxygen saturations consistent with previous data. Dashed vertical line marks pre-prediction and post-prediction time line. Blue shadow to the right of the vertical dashed line shows oxygen saturation data consistent with previously sampled data. Black line is actual oxygen saturation. Dashed blue line is expected average oxygen saturation.

Sensors Used in Continuous Monitoring

In the following paragraphs we review selected articles that used various sensors in the setting of continuous monitoring in GCUs. These sensors may monitor 1 or multiple physiologic variables that can be used for generating alerts. Criteria for being included in this overview were (1) automatically collected vital signs, (2) notification systems, (3) adequate sample size, and (4) use on GCUs. In addition to reported results, reported tolerance, and acceptance by patients is considered.

Single-sensor monitoring

Telemetry and electrocardiogram monitoring Remote electrocardiogram monitoring is currently of limited value in low-risk populations due to artifacts, tethering, and the difficulties with automated waveform interpretation when used as a continuous monitor. Concern about low value in low-risk patients,[28] cost,[29] and unneeded interventions[30] with the use of telemetry has prompted many institutions to limit use. Daily cost for a telemetry monitoring was estimated to be $1400 per day in 2009,[29] with few data to demonstrate benefit.[28] No studies with automated alerts in the GCU settings have been conducted.

Pulse oximetry Pulse oximetry generates several physiologic variables, of which some have been used in surveillance monitoring. When used as a surveillance monitor, the sensor is tolerated well by patients (more than 95%).[7,31] Using a pulse oximetry–based surveillance system with pager notification of nursing staff when alarm thresholds were crossed, Taenzer and colleagues[7] found a reduction of RRT alerts by 65% (**Fig. 4**) and a reduction of unplanned intensive care unit (ICU) transfers by more than 40% using a before-and-after study design with concurrent controls. The researchers found similar results when the same surveillance system was subsequently deployed on other postsurgical GCUs.[8] Alarm burden was 2 alerts per nurse covering 5 patients per shift or 0.08 alerts per day per bed. Cost saving opportunities based on reduction of unplanned ICU days estimated that implementation and hardware costs were recovered within the first year of use when reducing ICU days by approximately 150 days for a 36-patient unit.[8]

Of the physiologic parameters generated by the pulse oximetry sensor, only pulse rate and oxygen saturation have been investigated as a surveillance monitor, but

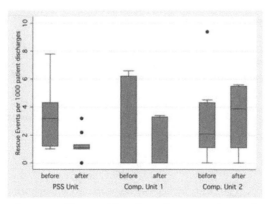

Fig. 4. Impact of patient surveillance with pulse oximetry on RRT activations per 1000 patient days contrasting the Patient Surveillance System (PSS) with 2 other surgical control units (CU). (*From* Taenzer AH, Pyke JB, McGrath SP, et al. Impact of pulse oximetry surveillance on rescue events and intensive care unit transfers: a before-and-after concurrence study. Anesthesiology 2010;112:282–87; with permission.)

not perfusion index, respiratory rate, or hemoglobin fractions. Pulse oximetry has high accuracy and precision, and artifacts are minimal, making it an ideal sensor suitable for continuous monitoring (**Box 1**).

Piezoelectric sensor Under-the-mattress, contactless, piezoelectric sensors have been used to monitor heart (HR) and respiratory rate (RR),[32] as well as patient's motion to alert when thresholds were crossed. In a before-and-after study design, a rate of 0.06 alerts per day per bed for HR and 0.3 alerts per day per bed for RR was found. Although transfers to the ICU did not change, length of stay (LOS) of those transferred decreased by approximately 50%, as did overall LOS in the postimplementation period.[33] Patients' tolerances can be assumed to be excellent, as this is a contactless sensor. Cost sensitivity analysis demonstrated that cost could be recuperated in the first year of use.[34]

Sound-based respiratory rate monitoring Acoustic-based RR monitoring has been shown to have modestly better precision and accuracy than capnometry for RR in postsurgical patients.[35] The sensor requires a sticker be placed on the patient's neck tethered via a cord to a monitor. In a postsurgical population, almost 20% of patients refused to be connected to the sensor.[27] When used in addition to an existing pulse oximetry surveillance system,[7,31] acoustic-based respiratory rate monitoring did not change RRT events or ICU transfers in almost 5000 patient days monitored before and after.[27]

Multisensor monitoring
Using cableless sensors with additional spot check monitors, Subbe and colleagues[36] used HR, RR, blood pressure, temperature, and pulse oximetry in addition to conscious state to calculate early warning scores and alert system-trained nurses and physicians. The patient cohort consisted of patients with acute emergencies only who were continuously monitored. RRT notifications increased by approximately

---

Box 1
Desirable characteristics of electronic monitoring systems

Accurate and precise

Sensitive and specific

Continuous

Ability to trend in real time

Does not hinder patient mobility or impair comfort

Multimodal (multiple parameters measured with selection options)

Automated alert/alarm with directed alerts to various levels of care providers

Cost-effective, adaptable, and upgradable

Integrates with electronic medical record and existing alert systems

Failure mode recognition (detects when it is not working)

Adaptable display modes (in room, mobile devices, workstation monitors, remote)

"Smart," self-learning, artificial intelligence

Adapted from DeVita MA, Smith GB, Adam SK, et al. Identifying the hospitalised patient in crisis'—a consensus conference on the afferent limb of rapid response systems. Resuscitation 2006;81:375–82; with permission.

25%, whereas mortality and cardiac arrests decreased, as did the severity of illness of those admitted to the ICU. Alarm burden to providers or patient tolerance were not reported.

ALARM MANAGEMENT

The Joint Commission recommends that hospitals educate staff on the operation of alarm systems and have policies in place on how to manage alarms.[37] As discussed previously, continuous monitoring is likely to be used to a greater degree in the GCU setting where the patient-to-nurse ratio is higher than in the intermediate or ICU setting and the potential exposure of nurses to clinical bedside alarms is higher. The frequency of alarms in ICUs has been reported to be between 1.6 and 14.7 alarms per hour, with false alarms or those not leading to an intervention being as common as 90%.[38] This alarm burden rate has raised significant concerns, leading to the Joint Commission recommendations. If one extrapolates these alarm rates from ICU nurses taking care of 1 or 2 patients to a floor nurse caring for many, it is easily recognizable that alarm management for continuous monitoring on GCUs is of key importance, as described by McGrath and colleagues.[25] Hence, reviewers and editors should mandate the reporting of alarm frequencies from researchers when reporting on continuous monitoring and as staffing ratios vary among institutions, these rates should be reported as alarms per bed per day.

DISCUSSION

Given that there are few published articles that meet the minimum criteria listed previously, one has to conclude that there is a paucity of data on the value of continuous monitoring.

The previously cited studies by Brown and colleagues,[33] Subbe and colleagues,[36] and Taenzer and colleagues,[7] have in common an implementation phase that included user education and a notification system. They also all had positive impacts on the outcome variables measured. It is desirable that studies do report on alarm burdens and strategies to mitigate them,[25] as well as on patient compliance and tolerance. Of the 3 studies discussed previously, only Brown and colleagues[33] and Taenzer and colleagues[7] reported on alarm frequencies, using different metrics. Although Brown and colleagues[33] did not report on patient acceptance, this can be implied to be superb, as they used a contactless sensor. Taenzer and colleagues[7] reported on acceptance rates of pulse oximeter probe, as well as the sound-based respiratory sensor.

Studying the reduction of rare events is difficult, and as Berwick argued in "The Science of Improvement,"[39] randomized controlled trials are ill suited to do so. Although randomized controlled trials may be criticized for generating results under conditions that will never be the same, they do generate solid evidence for targeted interventions, especially when environmental variables that cannot be randomized or controlled for have little impact on outcomes. When implementing complex interventions, such as introducing RRT or continuous monitoring in GCUs, one is essentially altering how the hospital functions. The target group for which outcomes are reported are not individuals, or groups of individuals that share a diagnosis, but rather patients who share a hospital location (ie, general care unit or orthopedic unit), as continuous monitoring would be rolled out by 1 or more unit. Hence, these interventions are not suitable for randomized (including cluster) controlled trials, but are better done using before-and-after study design, ideally using other units concurrently as controls.[7,33]

Although some health care systems, like the authors' hospital, have implemented hospital-wide continuous monitoring on GCUs since 2009, this has not become widespread practice. Dartmouth Hitchcock Medical Center requires patients to sign waivers if they request not to be monitored after being educated on the benefits of monitoring, along with the documentation of those wishes. The introduction of such continuous monitoring systems is a tremendous hospital-wide effort that is resource intensive. Primary barriers to adoption appear to be complexity, cost, and difficult-to-interpret medical evidence. As a significant portion of health care change is driven by economics, and therefore evolving reimbursement models that penalize for complications, extended periods of stay and readmissions may drive broader adoption, along with the ever-increasing acuity and comorbidity indices of those residing in hospitals. Health and vital sign monitoring seems to be becoming ubiquitous with the personal use of mobile device health care applications, and expectations, as well as acceptance, should drive in-hospital monitoring forward. The authors believe that the time to implement continuous monitoring on GCUs has arrived, and provides the basis for future developments, such as postdischarge and home monitoring.

REFERENCES

1. Taenzer AH, Pyke JB, McGrath SP. A review of current and emerging approaches to address failure-to-rescue. Anesthesiology 2011;115:421–31.
2. Kause J, Smith G, Prytherch D, et al. A comparison of antecedents to cardiac arrests, deaths and emergency intensive care admissions in Australia and New Zealand, and the United Kingdom–the ACADEMIA study. Resuscitation 2004; 62:275–82.
3. Bedell SE, Deitz DC, Leeman D, et al. Incidence and characteristics of preventable iatrogenic cardiac arrests. JAMA 1991;265:2815–20.
4. Schein RM, Hazday N, Pena M, et al. Clinical antecedents to in-hospital cardiopulmonary arrest. Chest 1990;98:1388–92.
5. DeVita MA, Braithwaite RS, Mahidhara R, et al, Medical Emergency Response Improvement Team (MERIT). Use of medical emergency team responses to reduce hospital cardiopulmonary arrests. Qual Saf Health Care 2004;13:251–4.
6. DeVita MA, Smith GB, Adam SK, et al. Identifying the hospitalised patient in crisis—a consensus conference on the afferent limb of rapid response systems. Resuscitation 2006;81:375–82.
7. Taenzer AH, Pyke JB, McGrath SP, et al. Impact of pulse oximetry surveillance on rescue events and intensive care unit transfers: a before-and-after concurrence study. Anesthesiology 2010;112:282–7.
8. Blike G, Taenzer AH. Postoperative monitoring-the Dartmouth experience. APSF Newsl 2010;27:1.
9. Overdyk FJ, Carter R, Maddox RR, et al. Continuous oximetry/capnometry monitoring reveals frequent desaturation and bradypnea during patient-controlled analgesia. Anesth Analg 2007;105:412–8.
10. HealthGrades Eighth Annual Patient Safety in American Hospitals Study. AHRQ Patient Safety Network. 2017. [Online]. Available: https://psnet.ahrq.gov/resources/resource/21246. Accessed April 15, 2017.
11. Hall MJ, Levant S, DeFrances CJ. Trends in inpatient hospital deaths: National Hospital Discharge Survey, 2000-2010. NCHS Data Brief 2013;118:1–8.
12. Mitchell I, Van Leuvan CH. Missed opportunities? An observational study of vital sign measurements. Crit Care Resusc 2004;10(2):111.

13. Abenstein JP, Narr BJ. An ounce of prevention may equate to a pound of cure. Anesthesiology 2008;112:272–3.
14. Gallagher SF, Haines KL, Osterlund LG, et al. Postoperative hypoxemia: common, undetected, and unsuspected after bariatric surgery. J Surg Res 2010; 159:622–6.
15. Taenzer AH, Pyke J, Herrick MD, et al. A comparison of oxygen saturation data in inpatients with low oxygen saturation using automated continuous monitoring and intermittent manual data charting. Anesth Analg 2014;118:326–31.
16. Sun Z, Sessler DI, Dalton JE, et al. Postoperative hypoxemia is common and persistent: a prospective blinded observational study. Anesth Analg 2015;121: 709–15.
17. Hooker EA, O'Brien DJ, Danzl DF, et al. Respiratory rates in emergency department patients. J Emerg Med 1987;7:129–32.
18. Villegas I, Arias IC, Botero A, et al. Evaluation of the technique used by healthcare workers for taking blood pressure. Hypertension 1995;26:1204–6.
19. Cardona-Morrell M, Prgomet M, Turner RM, et al. Effectiveness of continuous or intermittent vital signs monitoring in preventing adverse events on general wards: a systematic review and meta-analysis. Int J Clin Pract 2016;70:806–24.
20. Welch J, Kanter B, Skora B, et al. Multi-parameter vital sign database to assist in alarm optimization for general care units. J Clin Monit Comput 2016;30:895–900.
21. Hillman K. The changing role of acute-care hospitals. Med J Aust 1999;170(7): 325–8.
22. Le Maguet P, Roquilly A, Lasocki S, et al. Prevalence and impact of frailty on mortality in elderly ICU patients: a prospective, multicenter, observational study. Intensive Care Med 2014;40(5):674–82.
23. Yoder JC, Arora VM, Edelson DP. Acutely ill patients will likely benefit from more monitoring, not less–reply. JAMA Intern Med 2014;174(3):475–6.
24. Bellomo R, Ackerman M, Bailey M, et al. A controlled trial of electronic automated advisory vital signs monitoring in general hospital wards. Crit Care Med 2012; 40(8):2349–61.
25. McGrath SP, Taenzer AH, Karon N, et al. Surveillance monitoring management for general care units: strategy, design, and implementation. Jt Comm J Qual Patient Saf 2014;42:293–302.
26. Pyke J, Taenzer AH, Renaud CE, et al. Developing a continuous monitoring infrastructure for detection of inpatient deterioration. Jt Comm J Qual Patient Saf 2010; 38:428.
27. McGrath SP, Pyke J, Taenzer AH. Assessment of continuous acoustic respiratory rate monitoring as an addition to a pulse oximetry-based patient surveillance system. J Clin Monit Comput 2016;31(3):561–9.
28. Schull MJ, Redelmeier DA. Continuous electrocardiographic monitoring and cardiac arrest outcomes in 8,932 telemetry ward patients. Acad Emerg Med 2000; 7(6):647–52.
29. Henriques-Forsythe MN, Ivonye CC, Jamched U, et al. Is telemetry overused? Is it as helpful as thought? Cleve Clin J Med 2009;76(6):368–72.
30. Knight BP, Pelosi F, Michaud GF, et al. Clinical consequences of electrocardiographic artifact mimicking ventricular tachycardia. N Engl J Med 1999;341(17): 1270–4.
31. Taenzer A, Blike G. Postoperative surveillance—the Dartmouth experience. APSF Newsl 2010;27:1.
32. Ben-Ari J, Zimlichman E, Adi N, et al. Contactless respiratory and heart rate monitoring: validation of an innovative tool. J Med Eng Technol 2010;34(7–8):393–8.

33. Brown H, Terrence J, Vasquez P, et al. Continuous monitoring in an inpatient medical-surgical unit: a controlled clinical trial. Am J Med 2014;127:226–32.

34. Slight SP, Franz C, Olugbile M, et al. The return on investment of implementing a continuous monitoring system in general medical-surgical units. Crit Care Med 2014;42(8):1862–8.

35. Ramsay MAE, Usman M, Lagow E, et al. The accuracy, precision and reliability of measuring ventilatory rate and detecting ventilatory pause by rainbow acoustic monitoring and capnometry. Anesth Analg 2013;117(1):69–75.

36. Subbe CP, Duller B, Bellomo R. Effect of an automated notification system for deteriorating ward patients on clinical outcomes. Crit Care 2017;21:52.

37. The Joint Commission. 2016 comprehensive accreditation manual for hospitals (E-dition). Oak Brook (IL): Joint Commission; 2015.

38. Imhoff M, Kuhls S. Alarm algorithms in critical care monitoring. Anesth Analg 2006;102(5):1525–37.

39. Berwick D. The science of improvement. JAMA 2008;299:1182–4.

Trigger Criteria: Big Data

Kim Moi Wong Lama, MD[a],*, Michael A. DeVita, MD, FRCP[b,1]

KEYWORDS

- Rapid response system • Monitoring • Risk prediction • Deterioration

KEY POINTS

- The US health care system is rapidly adopting electronic medical records (EMRs). The capability to analyze a huge amount of clinical data during a care episode will dramatically increase.
- Existing analytical techniques can be applied to enable better prediction of outcomes, which can be applied to the point-of-care decision-making process.
- This change will occur in the near future.
- Aggregate warning systems for imminent death using vital sign abnormalities are now being combined with so-called big data derived from the EMR, offering a great opportunity to detect and respond to the clinical changes that precede clinical deterioration and rapid response team activation.

INTRODUCTION

The US health care system is rapidly adopting electronic medical records (EMRs) and this will dramatically increase the quantity of clinical data available for sophisticated analysis during inpatient and outpatient care. Outpatient information that is becoming routinely available includes notifications of when patients fill their prescriptions and when they use their devices, such as an inhaler for asthma or chronic obstructive pulmonary disease, and noninvasive positive pressure ventilators for obstructive sleep apnea, as well as compliance with follow-up in outpatient clinics. Inpatient data include recent laboratory tests, imaging, vital sign monitoring with continuous electrocardiogram, carbon dioxide monitoring, pulse oximeters, and motion sensors that will monitor respiratory patterns and change in pulse. An integrated approach to analyzing this information creates the opportunity to improve health care quality, distribute resources adequately, and decrease cost. The types and quantity of information

Disclosure Statement: Dr K.M. Wong Lama has nothing to disclose. Dr M.A. DeVita is Chief Medical Officer of EarlySense Inc, a continuous vital sign monitoring company.
[a] Department of Internal Medicine, Columbia College of Physicians and Surgeons, Harlem Hospital Center, 506 Lenox Avenue, Room 6110, Mural Pavillion, New York, NY 10037, USA;
[b] Critical Care, Harlem Hospital Center, 506 Lenox Avenue, Room 6110, Mural Pavillion, New York, NY 10037, USA
[1] 22 Wilson Avenue, Norwalk, CT 06853.
* Corresponding author.
E-mail address: KimMoi.WongLama@nychhc.org

Crit Care Clin 34 (2018) 199–207
https://doi.org/10.1016/j.ccc.2017.12.007
0749-0704/18/© 2017 Elsevier Inc. All rights reserved.

criticalcare.theclinics.com

available and the ability to analyze it in ways that can affect patient management in real time are referred to as big data.

In 2012, big data was described as "large volumes of high velocity, complex and variable data that requires advanced techniques and technologies to enable the capture, storage, distribution, management and analysis of the information."[1] Existing analytical techniques can be applied to the vast amount of existing patient-related health and medical data to reach a deeper understanding of outcomes, which can be applied to point-of-care management and assist physicians and their patients during the decision-making process and help determine the most appropriate treatment option. Numerous questions can be addressed with big data analytics and the potential benefits include detecting diseases at earlier stages, managing specific individual and population health, and detecting health care fraud more quickly and efficiently.[2] Additionally, the McKinsey Global Institute estimates that big data analytics can generate more than $300 billion in savings in US health care through reduction of waste and inefficiency in clinical operations, research, and development.[3]

There are several opportunities to use big data to improve the quality of health care and decrease health care costs.[4] Some of these uses include

- Identification of high-cost patients
- Identification of patients at risk for readmission
- Triage of resources and estimation of the risk of complications for patients admitted to the hospital
- Early detection of clinical deterioration
- Identification of patients at risk for adverse effects from medications or treatment
- Identification and treatment optimization for diseases affecting multiple organs.

The applications of analysis of big data in health care are not limited to these examples. This is just the beginning of the growing list of benefits of data analysis in health care.

This article describes the potential impact of big data analysis on risk stratification and early detection of serious deterioration, including death. Although the application of big data analysis can affect care for a wide variety of syndromes and treatment modalities, this article focuses on the relationship between the ability to analyze huge data sets to identify and predict deterioration with the occurrence of clinical deterioration requiring a rapid response team (RRT) activation.

BIG DATA IN THE HOSPITAL WARDS

Sudden decompensation leading to cardiac arrest and death occurs uncommonly in hospital wards, affecting only about 1% of patients outside the intensive care unit (ICU). As much as 80% of cardiopulmonary arrests are preceded by prolonged periods of physiologic and clinical instability.[5] These signs may be present up to 24 hours before a serious clinical event requiring intensive interventions.[6] There are 2 approaches to determining when a crisis occurs that can be used as triggers for calling the RRT. The first is the single-parameter system. In this system, any single abnormal vital sign value that is out of bounds is sufficient for the rapid response system (RRS) to be activated. Although single-parameter systems have lower sensitivity and specificity than multiple-parameter and weighted systems, they are very easy to teach and implement. The other approach is to use an aggregate weighted scoring system (AWSS), the most common form of which is the early warning score (EWS) system and its many variants. EWS systems have been developed with the aim of identifying clinical deterioration early, have been recommended by the National Institution of Health and

Clinical Excellence,[7] and are mandated in some countries. In a review by Churpek and colleagues,[8] EWS systems were more accurate than other types of scoring systems for predicting cardiac arrest, mortality, ICU transfer, and a composite outcome. These include the VitalPAC EWS (ViEWS) system (VitalPac manufactured System Healthcare, London, UK) (**Table 1**), the standardized EWS system (**Table 2**), the modified EWS (MEWS) system (**Table 3**), and the cardiac arrest risk triage (CART) score (**Table 4**). An AWSS allocates points according to the degree of derangement of physiologic variables, which are combined to a composite score. The score is compared with predefined trigger thresholds and are used to direct a graded intervention response, such as increased vital signs monitoring and involvement of a medical emergency team (MET) or more experienced staff.[9]

The most common physiologic markers included in the AWSS are respiratory rate, oxygen saturation, systolic blood pressure, and temperature. Increased respiratory rate greater than 27 breaths per minute was a strong predictor of cardiopulmonary arrest in a study by Fieselmann and colleagues[10] that explored the vital signs 72 hours before cardiac arrest in 12 nonintensive care internal medicine units. In 2017, Mochizuki and colleagues[11] published a study that showed that an increased respiratory rate in an emergency department was as strong predictor of early clinical deterioration after discharge. Neurologic examination is also included; however, age is not commonly included. **Tables 1–3** show commonly used EWS systems.[12–14] They are sensitive and specific for detecting deterioration likely to proceed to death unless there is intervention to reverse the process.

In 2015, a study by Zadravecz and colleagues[15] showed that combining the Glasgow Coma Scale and the Richmond Agitation-Sedation Scale was more accurate than any scale alone or the criteria of alert, responds to voice, responds to pain, and unresponsive (AVPU) in predicting mortality. They proposed that routine tracking of these 2 scales may improve the accuracy of detecting clinical deterioration.

The EWS is not the only system for quantifying high-risk deterioration. There are several scoring scales developed to identify patients at risk for developing clinical decompensation, possible cardiac arrest and death. Some are single-parameter systems, such as the MET criteria reported by Hillman and colleagues.[16] These are the most simple to understand, teach, and implement; therefore, they are commonly used in hospitals even though they are less sensitive and specific than an AWSS, such as the MEWS system. The choice of the scoring system used for each hospital depends on their culture and resources.

Table 1 VitalPAC early warning score							
Score	3	2	1	0	1	2	3
Respiratory Rate	<9	—	9–11	11–20	—	21–24	>24
Oxygen Saturation	<92	92–93	94–95	96–100	—	—	—
Supplemental Oxygen	—	—	—	No	—	—	Yes
Heart Rate	—	<41	41–50	51–90	91–110	111–130	>130
Systolic BP	<91	91–100	101–110	111–249	>248	—	—
Temperature	<35.1	—	35.1–36	36.1–38	38.1–39	>39	—
Neurologic	—	—	—	Alert	—	—	Voice
	—	—	—	—	—	—	Pain
	—	—	—	—	—	—	Unresp

Abbreviations: BP, blood pressure; Unresp, unresponsive.

Table 2
Standardized early warning system

Score	3	2	1	0	1	2	3
Respiratory Rate	<8	—	—	9–20	21–30	31–35	>35
Oxygen Saturation	<85	85–89	90–92	>93	—	—	—
Heart Rate	<29	30–39	40–49	50–99	100–109	110–129	>129
Systolic BP	<69	70–79	80–99	100–199	—	>199	—
Temperature	<34	34–34.9	35–35.9	36–37.9	38–38.4	>38.4	—
Neurologic	Unresponsive	Pain	Verbal	Alert	—	—	—

BIG DATA, EVENT PREDICTION, AND EVENT DETECTION

The electronic medical record (EMR) and practical solutions to using it is quickly becoming available. Several researchers have created analytical programs for scanning the EMR to identify those at risk. The methodology used to create these systems vary; however, all access huge databases and use real-time data to generate a highly sensitive and specific risk score. The Worthington Physiologic Scoring System was derived from analysis of admission data, whereas the CART score was designed using logistic regression to detect in-hospital cardiac arrest and was validated for detecting ward-to-ICU transfers. The CART score performed better than the MEWS for detecting cardiac arrest and ICU transfer.[8] **Table 4** shows the CART scoring rubric.

The eCART system (Quant HC, Chicago, IL) goes further by using a broader data set. Kang and colleagues[17] designed a prospective black-box validation study, using real-time risk stratification with the eCART that incorporated laboratory information system, bedside patient monitor, and registration data into a scoring database through the integration engine. Patients were stratified as high risk or intermediate risk. The study demonstrated the feasibility of prospective real-time eCART calculation in a general ward and found that it detected 4 times as many cardiac arrests and 50% more ICU transfers compared with the current RRS to activate the RRT. In this study, eCART identified many high-risk patients who were missed by the current RRS using single-parameter triggers and, for those whom the RRT was called, identified those hours earlier.

Currently, the most common method to calculate scores in the AWSS is manual calculation, which can lead to calculation errors. Preprogrammed EMR or handheld device applications decrease errors in calculation but can be time-consuming and redundant to workflow. Ideally, a completed automated system integrated with the EMR and with automatic provider notification (nurse or physician, or even the MET) may be a more accurate and a less redundant way to apply the AWSS in the hospital wards.[9] These scoring systems may be considered small data because they use only a

Table 3
Modified early warning score

Score	3	2	1	0	1	2	3
Respiratory Rate	—	<9	—	9–14	15–20	21–29	>29
Heart Rate	—	<40	41–50	51–100	101–110	111–129	>129
Systolic BP	<70	71–80	81–100	101–199	—	>199	—
Temperature	—	<35	—	35–38.4	—	>38.4	—
Neurologic	—	—	—	Alert	Voice	Pain	Unresp

Table 4	
Cardiac arrest risk triage score	
Vital Sign	**Score**
Respiratory Rate, breaths/min	
<21	0
21–23	8
24–25	12
26–29	15
>29	22
Heart Rate, beats/min	
<110	0
110–39	4
>139	13
Diastolic BP, mm Hg	
>49	0
40–49	4
35–39	6
<35	13
Age, years	
<55	0
55–69	4
>69	9

small portion of the data that exist about a patient to create a risk score. So-called big data, in contrast, can access a virtually unbounded data set, including medications, prior hospitalizations, genetic phenotype, age, sex, laboratory and imaging data, social habits, and other indices, such as a frailty index.

There is a significant debate about which approach is better. Single-parameter scores are easier, whereas aggregate weighted scores have better sensitivity and specificity. Mohammed and colleagues[18] showed that, as the EWS increases, the probability of a calculation error goes up, making the EWS system less attractive. However, there are now several options for calculating the EWS in an automated fashion, making the task simpler, faster, and more accurate. Hand-held computer help to improve the accuracy and efficiency of EWS systems in acute hospital care is acceptable to nurses. Hospitals that have fully capable EMRs can incorporate more complex algorithms, including results of laboratory studies. EMR-based detection of impending deterioration outside the ICU is feasible and can reach its maximal potential in integrated health care delivery systems that provide access to outpatient data, such as physician office records, rehabilitation notes, skilled nursing facility visits, and pharmacy records.[19] The potential is still being ascertained; however, many providers are very optimistic about the ability of these analytics not only to predict immediate risk of death but also to facilitate diagnosis of a variety of ailments.

MEDICAL EMERGENCY TEAMS AND RISK STRATIFICATION OF HOSPITALIZED PATIENTS

Identifying the patients at risk for clinical deterioration and impending decompensation is only the first, but important, step. Once the patients are identified, mobilization

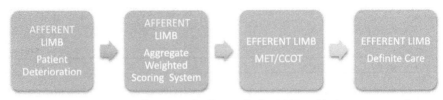

Fig. 1. RRS incorporation afferent and efferent limb. CCOT, critical care outreach team. (*From* DeVita MA, Braithwaite RS, Mahidhara R, et al. Medical Emergency Response Improvement Team (MERIT).Use of medical emergency team responses to reduce hospital cardiopulmonary arrests. Qual Saf Health Care 2004;13(4):251–4; with permission.)

of resources can be activated and deployed, such as METs and critical outreach teams.[20] The transfer to ICU, escalation of care to more monitored settings, or decompensation followed by cardiac arrest may not always be preventable; however, there will be an anticipated transition of care as opposed to emergent care. **Fig. 1** shows the integration between the afferent and efferent limbs of a MET.

Box 1
Clinical criteria for activating the medical emergency team

Respiration
- Rate less than 8 or greater than 36
- New onset of difficulty breathing
- New pulse oximeter reading less than 85% for more than 5 minutes (unless patient known to have chronic hypoxemia)

Heart rate
- Less than 40 or greater than 140 with symptoms
- Any greater than 160

Blood pressure
- Less than 80 or greater than 200 systolic blood pressure with symptoms
- Greater than 110 diastolic blood pressure with symptoms

Acute neurologic changes
- Acute loss of consciousness
- New onset lethargy or Narcan use without immediate response
- Seizure (outside of seizure monitor unit)
- Sudden loss of movement (or weakness) of face, arm, or leg

Other
- Chest pain, unresponsive to nitroglycerine or doctor unavailable
- Color change (of patient or extremity): pale, dusky gray, or blue
- Unexplained agitation more than 10 minutes
- Suicide attempt
- Uncontrolled bleeding

Data from Huh JW, Lim CM, Koh Y, et al. Activation of a medical emergency team using an electronic medical recording-based screening system*. Crit Care Med 2014;42(4):801–8.

A review by McNeill and Bryden,[21] published in *Resuscitation* in 2013, presented strong evidence that a MET improved hospital mortality, reduced unplanned ICU admissions, and reduced cardiac arrests. The AWSS also improved hospital survival and reduced both unplanned ICU admissions and cardiac arrest rates.

An AWSS triggering activation of a MET offers added benefits to the hospitalized patient with impending clinical decline.[21] Adopting an early AWSS may decrease the delay in the activation of a MET, which is a strong predictor of mortality.[22,23]

The clinical criteria for activating a MET offers a list of clinical changes as signs of clinical deterioration that will prompt MET activation (**Box 1**). In 2014, a randomized study by Kollef and colleagues[24] showed that real-time alerts triggered by early warning system and sent to the RRT before MET criteria was met did not reduce ICU transfers, hospital mortality, and/or the need for subsequent long-term care; however, length of stay in the hospital was modestly reduced. A modified MET was studied by Huh and colleagues,[25] which they used as a triggering tool for MET activation, that included screening criteria from the EMR (**Box 2**). The afferent limb and the activation of a MET could be triggered by EMR-based screening or by a call from a bedside medical team. The efferent limb included physicians, nurses, and respiratory therapists who were responsible for providing early goal-directed therapy for shock, respiratory care (eg, advanced airway management), and cardiopulmonary

---

Box 2
Triggering tool for medical emergency activation team

Screening criteria from EMR
  Systolic mean blood pressure less than 60 mm Hg or systolic blood pressure less than 90 mm Hg
  Respiratory distress (rate >25 or <8 breaths per minute)
  Unexplained pulse rate greater than 130 beats per minute or pulse rate less than 50 beats per minute
  Unexplained metabolic acidosis (pH <7.3) or lactate greater than 2 mmol per liter
  $Paco_2$ greater than 50 mm Hg or Pao_2 less than 55 mm Hg
  Glucose less than 2.8 mmol per liter
  Sudden mental status changes or unexplained agitation
  Applying oxygen nasal prong greater than 3 L, or Venturi mask greater than 30%
  Unexplained seizures
  Chest pain
  Upper airway obstruction sign: stridor

Calling criteria
  Airway
  • Threatened
  • Stridor
  Breathing
  • Respiratory rate less than 6 breaths per minute
  • Respiratory rate greater than 30 breaths per minute
  • SpO_2 less than 90% on Venturi mask 40% or oxygen 12 L per minute
  Circulation
  • Pulse rate less than 40 beats per minute
  • Pulse rate greater than 140 beats per minute
  • Systolic blood pressure less than 90 mm Hg
  Neurology
  • Sudden mental change
  • Seizure
  Others
  • Bedside nurse's concern about overall deterioration

Cardiopulmonary resuscitation code blue

resuscitation. The EMR-triggered group had lower ICU admissions than the call-triggered group.

There is significant variability in the availability of data, the EMR, and resources in each hospital system. Adopting an early warning system and integrating this with the EMR with real-time communication to a fully staffed MET may be the ultimate goal to decrease the number of cases with acute decompensation that occur in the inpatient wards. Further studies and description of the requirements are needed.

SUMMARY

Aggregate warning systems, in combination with big data derived from the EMR, offers a great opportunity to detect clinical changes that precede a MET activation. Further studies are needed to determine if this will decrease the number of transfers to the ICU and cardiac arrests on the floors, as well as improve outcomes. Data interpretation depends significantly on the EMR available in each hospital and the resources available at each site. This variability affects both the afferent and the efferent limbs of the medical emergency systems.

Real-time big data analytics have the potential to transform the way health care providers use technologies to gain insight from clinical and other data repositories and make informed decisions.[2] In the future, the authors expect the use of big data analytics, including an AWSS, will allow providers to predict that a patient will meet clinical criteria to activate MET and enable intervention before the critical moment happens. More research is needed to determine if this early identification will affect patient clinical outcomes, including cardiac arrest, transfer to the ICU, length of stay, morbidity, and mortality.

REFERENCES

1. Institute for Health Technology Transformation (IHTT). Transforming Health Care through Big Data Strategies for leveraging big data in healthcare care industry. 2013. Available at: http://c4fd63cb482ce6861463-bc6183f1c18e748a49b87a25911a0555. r93.cf2.rackcdn.com/iHT2_BigData_2013.pdf.
2. Raghupathi W, Raghupathi V. Big data analytics in healthcare: promise and potential. Health Inf Sci Syst 2014;2:3.
3. Manyika J, Chui M, Brown B, et al. Big data: the next frontier for innovation, competition, and productivity. New York: McKinsey Global Institute; 2011.
4. Bates DW, Saria S, Ohno-Machado L, et al. Big data in health care: using analytics to identify and manage high-risk and high-cost patients. Health Aff (Millwood) 2014;33(7):1123–31.
5. Galhotra S, DeVita MA, Simmons RL, et al, Members of the Medical Emergency Response Improvement Team (MERIT) Committee. Mature rapid response system and potentially avoidable cardiopulmonary arrests in hospital. Qual Saf Health Care 2007;16(4):260–5.
6. McGaughey J, Alderdice F, Fowler R, et al. Outreach and Early Warning Systems (EWS) for the prevention of intensive care admission and death of critically ill adult patients on general hospital wards. Cochrane Database Syst Rev 2007;(3):CD005529.
7. National Institute of Health and Clinical Excellence. Acutely ill patients in hospital: recognition of and response to acute illness in adults in hospital. London: National Institute of Health and Clinical Excellence; 2007. NICE Clinical Guideline No. 50.
8. Churpek MM, Yuen TC, Edelson DP. Risk stratification of hospitalized patients on the wards. Chest 2013;143(6):1758–65.

9. Jansen JO, Cuthbertson BH. Detecting critical illness outside the ICU: the role of track and trigger systems. Curr Opin Crit Care 2010;16(3):184–90.

10. Fieselmann JF, Hendryx MS, Helms CM. Respiratory rate predicts cardiopulmonary arrest for internal medicine inpatients. J Gen Intern Med 1993;8(7):354–60.

11. Mochizuki K, Shintani R, Mori K, et al. Importance of respiratory rate for the prediction of clinical deterioration after emergency department discharge: a single-center, case-control study. Acute Med Surg 2016;4(2):172–8.

12. Prytherch DR, Smith GB, Schmidt PE, et al. ViEWS–Towards a national early warning score for detecting adult inpatient deterioration. Resuscitation 2010;81(8):932–7.

13. Paterson R, MacLeod DC, Thetford D, et al. Prediction of in-hospital mortality and length of stay using an early warning scoring system: clinical audit. Clin Med 2006;6(3):281–4.

14. Subbe CP, Kruger M, Rutherford P. Validation of a modified early warning score in medical admissions. QJM 2001;94(10):521–6.

15. Zadravecz FJ, Tien L, Robertson-Dick BJ, et al. Comparison of mental-status scales for predicting mortality on the general wards. J Hosp Med 2015;10(10):658–63.

16. Hillman K, Chen J, Cretikos M, et al. Introduction of the medical emergency team (MET) system: a cluster-randomised controlled trial. Lancet 2005;365:2091–7.

17. Kang MA, Churpek MM, Zadravecz FJ, et al. Real-time risk prediction on the wards: a feasibility study. Crit Care Med 2016;44(8):1468–73.

18. Mohammed M, Hayton R, Clements G, et al. Improving accuracy and efficiency of early warning scores in acute care. Br J Nurs 2009;18(1):18–24.

19. Escobar GJ, LaGuardia JC, Turk BJ, et al. Early detection of impending physiologic deterioration among patients who are not in intensive care: development of predictive models using data from an automated electronic medical record. J Hosp Med 2012;7(5):388–95.

20. DeVita MA, Bellomo R, Hillman K, et al. Findings of the first consensus conference on medical emergency teams. Crit Care Med 2006;34(9):2463–78.

21. McNeill G, Bryden D. Do either early warning systems or emergency response teams improve hospital patient survival? A systematic review. Resuscitation 2013;84(12):1652–67.

22. Calzavacca P, Licari E, Tee A, et al. The impact of rapid response system on delayed emergency team activation patient characteristics and outcomes–a follow-up study. Resuscitation 2010;81(1):31–5.

23. Calzavacca P, Licari E, Tee A, et al. A prospective study of factors influencing the outcome of patients after a Medical Emergency Team review. Intensive Care Med 2008;34(11):2112–6.

24. Kollef MH, Chen Y, Heard K, et al. A randomized trial of real-time automated clinical deterioration alerts sent to a rapid response team. J Hosp Med 2014;9(7):424–9.

25. Huh JW, Lim CM, Koh Y, et al. Activation of a medical emergency team using an electronic medical recording-based screening system*. Crit Care Med 2014;42(4):801–8.

Surgical Rescue in Medical Patients

The Role of Acute Care Surgeons as the Surgical Rapid Response Team

Alexandra Briggs, MD[a], Andrew B. Peitzman, MD[b],*

KEYWORDS

- Surgical rescue • Surgical rapid response • Emergency surgery • Failure to rescue

KEY POINTS

- Surgical rescue is defined by the assessment and operative management required to prevent death in a critically ill patient.
- Failure to rescue occurs as a result of both microsystem and macrosystem factors, which encompass elements of both individual and hospital system performance.
- Partnership between medical and surgical providers is essential for the timely diagnosis and management of surgical pathology in the medical intensive care unit.

INTRODUCTION

Ward patients may deteriorate insidiously to the point of cardiopulmonary arrest. This clinical decline, on average over 6 hours, is often not recognized and frequently preventable. Rapid response systems have developed as a means to promptly provide a team to intervene and abort the downhill spiral. There are 4 elements to this response, as described in the First Consensus Conference on Medical Emergency Teams: the afferent component during which the patient is identified and the team activated; the efferent component, during which the response team provides the expertise for intervention; the process improvement component, which provides ongoing quality evolution; and the administrative component, which creates organizational and educational structure.[1] The criteria that precipitate activation generally include thresholds for heart rate, blood pressure, and mental status, as well as "gut feeling" of the staff.[2,3] The inciting complications are usually medical and include pulmonary embolism, myocardial infarction, dysrhythmia, pneumonia, stroke, sepsis, and respiratory

[a] Department of Surgery, University of Pittsburgh, F-1281, UPMC-Presbyterian, Pittsburgh, PA 15213, USA; [b] Department of Surgery, University of Pittsburgh School of Medicine, F-1281, UPMC-Presbyterian, Pittsburgh, PA 15213, USA
* Corresponding author.
E-mail address: peitzmanab@upmc.edu

Crit Care Clin 34 (2018) 209–219
https://doi.org/10.1016/j.ccc.2017.12.002
0749-0704/18/© 2017 Elsevier Inc. All rights reserved.

criticalcare.theclinics.com

fatigue. Although the incipient complication may not be preventable, further deterioration and death often are avoidable if promptly identified and the appropriate response team activated. In the surgical population, complications are 2 to 4 times more common compared with medical patients, despite only 40% of in-hospital complications being due to surgical procedures. Surgical complications are more likely to be avoidable (from operative error), with more serious consequences of the surgical complication; such as common bile duct injury during cholecystectomy or anastomotic leak after a bowel resection. After a complication has occurred, the goal of the clinical care team is to prevent further deterioration, additional complications, and at the most extreme, death, which would be defined as *failure to rescue*.[4] Prompt intervention and salvage of the patient after a surgical (operative or interventional) complication is defined as *surgical rescue*.[5] In the medical population, this concept of rescue also can be applied to the 2% to 4% of intensive care unit (ICU) patients who will require surgical intervention for intra-abdominal pathology. The most frequent indications for abdominal operation in ICU patients are bowel perforation, bowel ischemia, cholecystitis, bowel obstruction or volvulus, and severe *Clostridium difficile* colitis (**Box 1**).[6,7]

Surgical rescue has recently developed as an essential part of acute care surgery practice, as surgeons have become increasingly involved in emergency interventions for critically ill patients.[5,8–10] Analysis of Centers for Disease Control and Prevention (CDC) discharge data shows that 41% of all hospital discharges are emergent, and 25% are urgent, demonstrating the overall high acuity of the care we provide. Further evaluation of the CDC data reveals that more than 1 million patient discharges are a result of "surgical and medical complications," greater than the number discharges for the common medical admission diagnoses of septicemia, diabetes, or bronchitis.[11] A review of the experience in our own institution noted that 13% (320 of 2410) of our acute care surgery patients were treated for procedural complications; 85% were postoperative, but notably with 15% related to interventional or endoscopic procedures. These patients are acutely ill, 49% requiring ICU admission, and 63% requiring operative intervention. The care required for the survival of these patients necessitates the teamwork of multiple surgical subspecialties and interventionalists, support from intensivists through the management of mechanical ventilation, vasopressor and nutritional support, and careful monitoring for additional complications. All of these teams and resources represent the "efferent limb" of an institutional rapid response system (RRS), each providing an area of expertise critical to the care of the patient. *Surgical*

Box 1
Abdominal catastrophes in the intensive care unit

Mesenteric ischemia

Perforated ulcer

Acute cholecystitis

Pancreatitis

Clostridium difficile colitis

Bowel obstruction

Abdominal compartment syndrome

Massive gastrointestinal bleeding

Ruptured visceral or aortic aneurysm

rescue most directly refers to the operative intervention and expertise required to save these patients from a poor outcome, and in the context of the larger RRS, the surgical team therefore acts as a "surgical rapid response team." Deficits at an individual or institutional level, or breakdown of any portion of the RRS can lead to *failure to rescue*. This article focuses on events in which surgical rescue is required in the medical patient, the themes of rescue (and failure to rescue), and the importance of partnership between medical and surgical providers to promptly and successfully care for our shared patients.

FAILURE TO RESCUE: PRINCIPLES AND APPLICATIONS TO THE MEDICAL POPULATION

In 1992, Silber and colleagues[4] published the seminal work defining "failure to rescue" as "death after an adverse occurrence." This initial publication analyzed complications after surgical procedures and noted that both patient and hospital factors contributed to complications and deaths. Much of the subsequent literature has focused on failure to rescue in a surgical population, to determine why patients die after operation, from predominantly medical complications, such as myocardial infarction, pulmonary embolism, pneumonia, or stroke. Multiple large-scale analyses have shown that differences in outcomes between low-performing and high-performing (or low and high volume) hospitals are related to failure to rescue rates rather than complication rates.[12,13] This suggests that there are factors at the hospital level that differentiate between successful and unsuccessful management of similar complications. It should also be noted that each additional complication suffered by a patient confers increased risk of failure to rescue, indicating that these patients are vulnerable to further deterioration once an initial insult has occurred and therefore must be promptly managed.[14,15] To rescue patients, we must understand the factors that contribute to our failures, both on an individual and system level. Recent literature on failure to rescue classifies these as macrosystem factors, such as hospital technology, resources, and staffing ratios, and microsystem factors, such as ICU and rapid response team composition, along with hospital culture, both at the institutional and individual levels.[16–23]

The sources of failure to rescue are not yet well defined, specifically in the combined medical/surgical population. The microsystem and macrosystem causes of failure to rescue that are seen in the surgical literature are likely to be applicable to the shared medical patient who requires surgical intervention. In medical ICU (MICU) patients undergoing surgery for abdominal pathology, Kollef and Allen[6] discovered multiple physiologic differences between survivors and nonsurvivors, including Acute Physiology and Chronic Health Evaluation (APACHE II) scores and severity of organ dysfunction. However, they also determined that there was a higher rate of diagnostic delay in nonsurvivors compared with survivors: 71.4% versus 9.5%. This raises the question of whether cognitive errors may be particularly important in the management of medical patients with surgical problems. Gajic and colleagues[7] also analyzed factors contributing to mortality rates in MICU patients undergoing surgery for abdominal diagnoses, again finding that physiologic factors, such as renal insufficiency and APACHE (III) scores, were associated with mortality, as was a diagnosis of ischemic bowel. In addition, delay in surgical evaluation and intervention was found to be significantly associated with mortality. A subanalysis demonstrated that risk factors for surgical delay included opiate and antibiotic use, altered mental status and mechanical ventilation, and lack of peritoneal signs. Furthermore, the investigators determined that 53% of patients were initially misdiagnosed. These findings corroborate that cognitive and diagnostic errors directly contribute to failure to rescue these patients. In the context of the RRS structure, these deficits are failures in the afferent limb, which then cause delays in the efferent limb activation of the rapid response team and predispose the patient to further deterioration.

The role of diagnostic errors in medicine has been an ongoing subject of research over the past few decades.[24,25] In a 2002 review, Graber and colleagues[26] divided diagnostic errors into 3 categories: no-fault errors, system errors, and cognitive errors. Failures in the diagnosis of critically ill medical patients may be due to a combination of each of these types of errors, and are related to the performance of both the individuals caring for the patient, as well as the larger hospital system. Although no-fault errors provide little opportunity for improvement, the system and cognitive errors are important to analyze to prevent or mitigate future faults. Hospitals often focus on technologic advancements, clinical and administrative oversight, and system-wide changes to combat these errors. Cognitive errors on the part of the individual have also been well described, and have resulted in the development of strategies to combat the bias and knowledge gaps that can result in these failures.[27] Surgical rescue in the MICU population requires significant clinical suspicion of surgical pathology by the medical team, with prompt consultation of the surgical team. The diagnosis must then be verified and the appropriate surgical management pursued. Each of these steps confers a risk of diagnostic error that could result in failure to rescue the patient. Another element of this process is the appropriate escalation of care (communication) when caregivers are concerned about the clinical status of the patient. Prior studies have demonstrated that failures can occur at each of 3 steps required during this process: identification of change in patient status, prompt communication to senior staff, and implementation of treatment.[21,22] When both medical and surgical teams are involved in patient care, escalation of care may be required within each team, again conferring risk of delay and subsequent failure to rescue. It is essential that both surgical and medical practitioners work to avoid both cognitive and communication failures to provide the best possible care to the patient.

SURGICAL RESCUE IN MEDICAL PATIENTS

Although the original concept of surgical rescue referred to the management of postoperative or postprocedural complications, the theme of rescue extends also to the emergency management of medical patients with surgical pathology. A subset of these patients is actively being treated in the MICU at the time of identification of a surgical disease that requires intervention. Kollef and Allen[6] studied more than 1600 consecutive admissions to a MICU and determined that 4.1% were diagnosed with abdominal pathology that could be addressed with surgery. The diverse array of diagnoses in these patients included bowel obstruction, intestinal ischemia, and perforation, along with biliary disease, gastrointestinal bleeding, and other conditions. Significant mortality was noted in these patients, with death in 100% of the patients who deferred surgery, whereas 25% of patients who had surgery subsequently died. A retrospective study of abdominal pathology in MICU patients at a single center found that 1.3% of patients admitted had an "acute abdominal catastrophe." Again, significant mortality was noted in this population, with 100% mortality in the patients who did not undergo surgery, and 44% mortality in those who underwent operation.[7] These studies demonstrate that although a small percentage of MICU patients develop abdominal pathology amenable to surgical intervention, these critically ill patients have high risk of mortality. These patients require prompt identification and management to rescue them from these surgical diseases; delay to operation results in avoidable mortality. Consultation of the acute care surgery service in the care of a critically ill medical patient can be considered as the activation of a surgical RRS to aid with rescue. After assessing the patient, the surgical team can provide guidance to aid with diagnosis, discussion of pathology with the patient and with family members, and surgical intervention when indicated.

SURGICAL PATHOLOGY IN MEDICAL PATIENTS

Patients on the inpatient medical service and in the MICU often have a complex set of comorbidities and acute disease processes that must be managed during the hospital stay. Identifying pathology that requires surgical intervention can sometimes be difficult in the setting of a complicated overall clinical scenario. Here we discuss some of the challenging diagnoses that require prompt identification and surgical management for successful rescue. These include medical pathology, such as abdominal compartment syndrome, severe *Clostridium difficile* infection, mesenteric ischemia, and massive bleeding, along with postprocedural complications from lines, tubes, and other invasive therapy.

Intra-abdominal hypertension (IAH) and abdominal compartment syndrome (ACS) are diagnoses often discussed in critically ill patients in the ICU. However, diagnosis and management of these conditions can be challenging. ACS is defined as primary ACS from an abdominal or pelvic process, versus secondary ACS from a nonabdominal or pelvic origin. A 2013 review separated risk factors for these processes into 3 broad categories: patient characteristics, systemic physiology, and fluid resuscitation. Factors that were common across multiple patient populations included respiratory status, large-volume crystalloid resuscitation, and shock.[28] Given that these factors are present in many of our ICU patients, it is important to know how to diagnose IAH and ACS. According to World Society of ACS guidelines, sustained or repeat bladder pressure measurements higher than 12 mm Hg are consistent with IAH, whereas ACS is characterized by measurements greater than 20 mm Hg in conjunction with organ dysfunction.[29] Management of IAH and ACS has been debated in the literature over recent years, particularly in patients with acute pancreatitis, with no clear consensus regarding the role for decompressive laparotomy versus medical or less invasive therapy in these patients.[30,31] However, the 2013 World Society of ACS guidelines do recommend decompressive laparotomy in cases of overt ACS, whether it is primary or secondary ACS.[29] Given that critically ill patients are at risk for the development of IAH and ACS, clinicians must be diligent to monitor for these processes in patients with multiple risk factors or diagnoses commonly associated with ACS. Involvement of a surgeon is reasonable when there is suspicion for IAH and ACS, for although there are methods for medical management of intra-abdominal pressure, a multidisciplinary approach helps to promptly identify and treat patients who need surgical decompression.

Clostridium difficile–associated disease (CDAD) is another common diagnosis that requires comanagement by medical and surgical teams. A recent review provided an overview of this increasingly common diagnosis, and reported that more than 9% of hospital admissions for these infections result in death. Options for medical management of these patients continue to expand with the use of new antibiotics, antibody therapy, and fecal microbiota transplantation.[32] However, a subset of these patients will develop severe or fulminant disease, which is associated with significant morbidity and mortality. Traditionally, surgical management of these patients required total colectomy, with approximately 1% of all patients with CDAD requiring this intervention.[33–35] Mortality rates for emergent colectomy have ranged between 30% and 80% and have been associated with a variety of preoperative physiologic factors and patient characteristics.[33–40] Interestingly, the duration of preoperative medical therapy has been associated with increased mortality,[33,34] whereas one study demonstrated that admission to a surgical department resulted in higher rates of operative intervention, shorter time to intervention, and decreased mortality.[36] Given that the optimal timing and patient selection for surgical therapy is not always evident, involvement of a surgeon is essential in patients with severe disease, or those who fail to have timely resolution of symptoms.[32] Communication between medical and surgical services is essential to promptly identify those patients who have worsening symptoms and require intervention. This can be achieved through a combination of institutional and departmental initiatives, including the adoption of protocols that mandate the involvement of the surgical team in the management of all patients with moderate or severe CDAD or provide specific criteria for consultation, and through outreach by surgeons to educate colleagues regarding identification and management of these infections. A culture of collegiality and openness between the medical and surgical services is also vital to promoting dialogue between teams for the benefit of patient care.

Acute mesenteric ischemia is an uncommon diagnosis that can be difficult to detect in the critically ill patient, but that carries mortality up to 90%.[41–45] In one large multicenter study of 780 patients in the ICU with mesenteric ischemia, the overall mortality rate was 58%, with increased mortality noted in older patients and those with higher organ failure scores. Notably, in this series, initial surgical intervention was one factor associated with decreased mortality. Only 14% of patients with nonoperative management survived.[41] A 2009 retrospective cohort study analyzing patient outcomes discovered that delay in operative management was associated with increased mortality, as were delays in surgical consultation and intervention in patients who did not have care withdrawn.[42] Another study demonstrated in univariate analysis that delay to surgery was associated with mortality.[43] It can be challenging to diagnose mesenteric ischemia, particularly in critically ill patients with numerous comorbidities, given the variability in clinical presentation, laboratory results, and imaging reliability. If there is clinical suspicion for mesenteric ischemia, early involvement of the surgical service is essential to aid with evaluation and management (**Fig. 1**). Compared with management of CDAD, it would be more difficult to protocolize consultation for this disease process given that there are not firm criteria for diagnosis. However, educational programs, such as combined medical and surgical conferences to discuss the topic of mesenteric ischemia, can provide valuable insight for both teams regarding recognition and management of this disease state. Furthermore, these sessions can serve to familiarize teams with one another and promote conversation between medical and surgical specialties.

Massive bleeding occurs in a variety of contexts in the ICU, and can lead to devastating outcomes if not promptly managed. Brisk gastrointestinal bleeding in ICU patients requires aggressive resuscitation and workup to identify and control the source. Although many of these patients can now be managed through the intervention of gastroenterologists and interventional radiologists, cases of refractory or unstable bleeding may require operative intervention for control. Early surgical consultation in patients with significant transfusion requirements, brisk bleeding, or hemodynamic instability is essential to achieve timely operative intervention, should other attempts at control not be feasible or are unsuccessful.[46–48]

Major arterial or venous bleeding can occur at access sites or after vascular operations, and can manifest as massive blood loss from such sites as the carotid or femoral vessels. At the first sign of an expanding hematoma or pulsatile bleeding, an attempt should be made to control the hemorrhage with direct compression at the site while emergent surgical consultation is obtained. In this situation, vascular

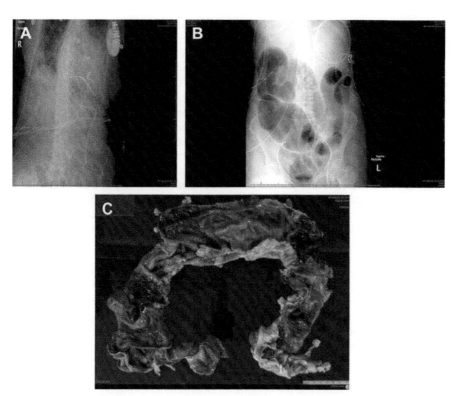

Fig. 1. A 67-year-old with a complicated cardiac history underwent mitral and tricuspid valvuloplasty 5 days before our consultation. The patient developed acute abdominal distension the morning on which we were consulted. He was hypotensive and on vasopressor support, afebrile, unreliable abdominal examination, distended, and tympanitic. Laboratory tests: white blood cell count 10,400/mm³, pH 7.43, HCO3 25, lactate 3.2 mMol/L. (*A*) Abdominal radiograph 24 hours to consultation. No free air, no air fluid levels. (*B*) Abdominal radiograph the morning of consultation. No free air, massive colonic distension. We presumed the acute abdominal distension and radiographic findings were from colonic ischemia: direct to the operating room. (*C*) Total colectomy was performed for diffuse colonic ischemia. The patient recovered.

access with large-bore intravenous or intraosseous lines and early transfusion is also essential. Another rare but catastrophic source of life-threatening bleeding occurs with tracheo-innominate fistula, which can be seen in the patient with a tracheostomy. This patient requires emergent surgical consultation and operative intervention, but control must be gained promptly to prevent death in the interim. At the bedside, over-inflation of the tracheostomy cuff can successfully contain bleeding in many cases. More invasive management options include direct digital compression of the innominate artery through the incision site after establishment of a distal airway, although it would be preferable to have surgical colleagues available for such a maneuver.[49] In all of these situations, the medical team must initiate resuscitation and attempt hemorrhage control, while quickly calling for the aid of surgical colleagues for definitive management.

Postprocedural complications also can require surgical evaluation and intervention in the medical ICU. These occur as misadventures of vascular access, or complications after endoscopic or interventional radiology procedures. One common source of clinical complications is gastrostomy tubes in patients requiring long-term enteral access. Complications of this procedure can occur at the time of placement, or can be discovered after prolonged use. These include transcolonic placement, which can cause early clinical decompensation or late identification of fistula development, abscess formation, buried bumper syndrome, or dislodgement of the tube.[50] Depending on the timing of these complications and the clinical status of the patient, some complications can require emergent operative intervention, whereas others can be managed at the bedside. Surgical consultation for evaluation of these patients is warranted whenever there is a concern about the position, appearance, or use of the tube so that appropriate management can be determined. Another procedure that is often performed in the ICU is colonoscopy, whether in the setting of gastrointestinal bleeding or workup for other pathologies. Although colonoscopy is a commonly performed and largely safe procedure, bowel perforation and splenic injury are rare but serious complications. Patients with hemodynamic instability or significant pain after colonoscopy should be evaluated promptly and surgical consultation should be obtained for aid with management.[51,52] These are just 2 examples of postprocedural complications that can arise in the ICU, and serve as a reminder that surgical consultation is always appropriate if there are concerns about a patient's condition.

Although the clinical scenarios described here represent only a fraction of those that require comanagement by medical and surgical practitioners, they are difficult to diagnose and triage in the critically ill patient. Medical providers must cultivate knowledge of the common and most life-threatening surgical processes in the ICU population, and be able to identify early warning signs of these conditions to allow early consultation and management by surgical colleagues. Similarly, surgeons must understand the altered physiology of these critically ill patients to make the correct diagnosis and determine the options for operative intervention.

A PARTNERSHIP FOR RESCUE

Surgical rescue is an evolving and essential part of surgery practice as we are confronted with numerous critically ill patients who require operative intervention. Although the concept of rescue often refers to the management required to overcome medical or surgical complications, it also can be extended to the management of surgical pathology in patients admitted to the medical service. These patients have significant comorbidity that makes them particularly vulnerable to clinical deterioration. At times, it can be difficult to promptly diagnose surgical diseases in the background of severe critical illness. Once a surgical problem is discovered, prompt consultation and management are required to rescue these patients from deterioration. Although we have discussed many factors that lead to rescue (or failure to rescue) in these patients, an essential element of rescue is teamwork among intensivists, hospitalists, and surgeons. Acute care surgeons are uniquely prepared to intervene in this population based on our daily practice, which is a combination of elective general surgery, surgical critical care, emergency general surgery, and trauma surgery. As a result, surgical rescue is now considered the "fifth pillar" of acute care surgery, drawing on expertise in the other 4 pillars of our specialty to intervene on patients who have suffered surgical complications or have developed surgical pathology during their hospitalization.[5] Acute care surgeons should be established as the surgical RRS for medical patients when the primary medical team is concerned about developing surgical pathology, and should be engaged as early as possible to aid with management. Interactions between surgical and medical services can be promoted through multiple initiatives, including the institution of protocols for surgical consultation for patients meeting specific criteria, and the creation of combined conferences between surgical and medical services on common surgical pathology seen by medical teams. Hospital and departmental leadership also must promote interactions among hospitalists, intensivists, and acute care surgeons so that practitioners at all levels feel comfortable initiating consults and providing recommendations for management. As we continue to define the needs of medical patients requiring surgical intervention, we all must work together to identify the challenges to patient care and overcome them to provide the optimal opportunity for rescue.

REFERENCES

1. DeVita MA, Bellomo R, Hillman K, et al. Findings of the first consensus conference on medical emergency teams. Crit Care Med 2006;34:2463–78.
2. Winters BD, Weaver SJ, Pfoh ER, et al. Rapid response systems as a patient safety strategy: a systematic review. Ann Int Med 2013;158:417–25.
3. Jones DA, DeVita MA, Bellomo R. Rapid response teams. N Engl J Med 2011; 365:139–46.
4. Silber JH, Williams SV, Krakauer H, et al. Hospital and patient characteristics associated with death after surgery. A study of adverse occurrence and failure to rescue. Med Care 1992;30:615–29.
5. Peitzman AB, Leppaniemi A, Kutcher ME, et al. Surgical rescue: an essential component of acute care surgery. Scand J Surg 2015;104:135–6.
6. Kollef MH, Allen BT. Determinants of outcome for patients in the medical intensive care unit requiring abdominal surgery. Chest 1994;106:1822–8.
7. Gajic O, Urrutia LE, Sewani H, et al. Acute abdomen in the medical intensive care unit. Crit Care Med 2002;30:1187–90.
8. Committee on Acute Care Surgery American Association for the Surgery of Trauma. The acute care surgery curriculum. J Trauma 2007;62(3):553–6.
9. Lewis AJ, Rosengart MR, Peitzman AB. Acute care surgery. In: Moore EE, Feliciano DV, Mattox KL, editors. Trauma. Philadelphia: McGraw-Hill; 2017. p. 97–102.
10. Kutcher ME, Sperry JL, Rosengart MR, et al. Surgical rescue: the next pillar of acute care surgery. J Trauma Acute Care Surg 2017;82(2):280–6.
11. Available at: http://www.cdc.gov/nchs/data.
12. Ghaferi AA, Birkmeyer JD, Dimick JB, et al. Complications, failure to rescue, and mortality with major inpatient surgery in Medicare patients. Ann Surg 2009;250: 1029–34.
13. Ghaferi AA, Birkmeyer JD, Dimick JB. Hospital volume and failure to rescue with high-risk surgery. Med Care 2011;49:1076–81.
14. Ferraris VA, Bolanos M, Martin JT, et al. Identification of patients with postoperative complications who are at risk for failure to rescue. JAMA Surg 2014;149(11): 1103–8.
15. Massarweh NN, Anaya DA, Kougias P, et al. Variation and impact of multiple complications on failure to rescue after inpatient surgery. Ann Surg 2017;266(1): 59–65.
16. Sheetz KH, Dimick JB, Ghaferi AA. Impact of hospital characteristics on failure to rescue following major surgery. Ann Surg 2016;263:692–7.
17. Aiken LH, Clarke SP, Sloane DM, et al. Hospital nurse staffing and patient mortality, nurse burnout and job dissatisfaction. JAMA 2002;288:1987–93.
18. Aiken LH, Clarke SP, Cheung RB, et al. Educational levels of hospital nurses and surgical patient mortality. JAMA 2003;290:1617–23.

19. Wakeam E, Hevelone ND, Maine R, et al. Failure to rescue in safety-net hospitals: availability of hospital resources and differences in performance. JAMA Surg 2014;149(3):229–35.
20. Ghaferi AA, Dimick JB. Importance of teamwork, communication and culture on failure-to-rescue in the elderly. Br J Surg 2016;103:e47–51.
21. Johnston M, Arora S, Anderson O, et al. Escalation of care in surgery: a systematic risk assessment to prevent avoidable harm in hospitalized patients. Ann Surg 2015;261(5):831–8.
22. Johnston MJ, Arora S, King D, et al. A systematic review to identify the factors that affect failure to rescue and escalation of care in surgery. Surgery 2015;157: 752–63.
23. Wakeam E, Asafu-Adjei D, Ashley SW, et al. The association of intensivists with failure to rescue rates in outlier hospitals: results of a national survey of intensive care unit organizational characteristics. J Crit Care 2014;29:930–5.
24. Brennan TA, Leape L, Laird N, et al. Incidence of adverse events and negligence in hospitalized patients: results of the Harvard Medical Practice Study I. N Engl J Med 1991;324:370–6.
25. Leape L, Brennan TA, Laird N, et al. The nature of adverse events in hospitalized patients: results of the Harvard Medical Practice Study II. N Engl J Med 1991;324: 377–84.
26. Graber M, Gordon R, Franklin N. Reducing diagnostic errors in medicine: what's the goal. Acad Med 2002;77:981–92.
27. Croskerry P. The importance of cognitive errors in diagnosis and strategies to minimize them. Acad Med 2003;78:775–80.
28. Holodinsky JK, Roberts DJ, Ball CG, et al. Risk factors for intra-abdominal hypertension and abdominal compartment syndrome among adult intensive care unit patients: a systematic review and meta-analysis. Crit Care 2013;17:R249.
29. Kirkpatrick AW, Roberts DJ, Waele JD, et al. Intraabdominal hypertension and the abdominal compartment syndrome: updated consensus definitions and clinical practice guidelines from the World Society of the Abdominal Compartment Syndrome. Intensive Care Med 2013;39:1190–206.
30. Radenkovic DV, Johnson CD, Milic N, et al. Interventional treatment of abdominal compartment syndrome during severe acute pancreatitis: current status and historical perspective. Gastroenterol Res Pract 2016;2016:5251806.
31. Mentula P, Hienonen P, Kemppainen E, et al. Surgical decompression for abdominal compartment syndrome in severe acute pancreatitis. Arch Surg 2010;145: 764–9.
32. Napolitano LM, Edmiston CE. Clostridium difficile disease: diagnosis, pathogenesis, and treatment update. Surgery 2017;162(2):325–48.
33. Halabi WJ, Nguyen VQ, Carmichael JC, et al. Clostridium difficile colitis in the United States: a decade of trends, outcomes, risk factors for colectomy, and mortality after colectomy. J Am Coll Surg 2013;2017:802–12.
34. Bryn JC, Maun DC, Gingold DS, et al. Predictors of mortality after colectomy for fulminant Clostridium difficile colitis. Arch Surg 2008;143:150–4.
35. Bhangu A, Nepogodiev D, Gupta A, et al, West Midlands Research Collaborative. Systematic review and meta-analysis of outcomes following emergency surgery for Clostridium difficile colitis. Br J Surg 2012;99:1501–13.
36. Sailhamer EA, Carson K, Chang Y, et al. Fulminant Clostridium difficile colitis: patterns of care and predictors of mortality. Arch Surg 2009;144:433–9.
37. Dudukgian H, Sie E, Gonzalez Ruiz C, et al. C. difficile colitis–predictors of fatal outcome. J Gastrointest Surg 2010;14:315–22.

38. Lee DY, Chung EL, Guend H, et al. Predictors of mortality after emergency colectomy for *Clostridium difficle* colitis: an analysis of ACS-NSQIP. Ann Surg 2015; 259:148–56.

39. Neal MD, Alverdy JC, Hall DE, et al. Diverting loop ileostomy and colonic lavage. Ann Surg 2011;254:423–9.

40. Fashandi AZ, Martin AN, Wang PT, et al. An institutional comparison of total abdominal colectomy and diverting loop ileostomy and colonic lavage in the treatment of severe, complicated *Clostridium difficile* infections. Am J Surg 2017;213:507–11.

41. Leone M, Bechis C, Baumstark K, et al. Outcome of acute mesenteric ischemia in the intensive care unit: a retrospective, multicenter study of 780 cases. Intensive Care Med 2015;41:667–76.

42. Eltarawy IG, Etman YM, Zenati M, et al. Acute mesenteric ischemia: the importance of early surgical consultation. Am Surg 2009;75:212–9.

43. Acosta-Merida MA, Marchena-Gomez J, Hemmersbach-Miller M, et al. Identification of risk factors for perioperative mortality in acute mesenteric ischemia. World J Surg 2006;30:1579–85.

44. Lee MJ, Sperry JL, Rosengart MR. Evaluating for acute mesenteric ischemia in critically ill patients: diagnostic peritoneal lavage is associated with reduced operative intervention and mortality. J Trauma Acute Care Surg 2014;77:441–7.

45. Gupta PK, Natarajan B, Gupta H, et al. Morbidity and mortality after bowel resection for acute mesenteric ischemia. Surgery 2011;150:779–87.

46. Strate LL, Gralnek IM. Management of patients with acute lower gastrointestinal bleeding. Am J Gastroenterol 2016;111:459–74.

47. Gerson LB, Fidler JL, Cave DR, et al. Diagnosis and management of small bowel bleeding. Am J Gastroenterol 2015;110:1265–87.

48. Raphaeli T, Menon R. Current treatment of lower gastrointestinal hemorrhage. Clin Colon Rectal Surg 2012;25:219–27.

49. Grant CA, Dempsey G, Harrison J, et al. Tracheo-innominate artery fistula after percutaneous tracheostomy: three case reports and a clinical review. Br J Anaesth 2006;96:127–31.

50. Schrag SP, Sharma R, Jaik NP, et al. Complications related to percutaneous endoscopic gastrostomy (PEG) tubes. A comprehensive clinical review. J Gastrointestin Liver Dis 2007;16:407–18.

51. Reumkens A, Randagh EJ, Bakker CM, et al. Post colonoscopy complications: a systematic review, time trends, and meta-analysis of population-based studies. Am J Gastroenterol 2016;111:1092–101.

52. Saad A, Rex DK. Colonoscopy-induced splenic injury: report of 3 cases and a literature review. Dig Dis Sci 2008;53:892–8.

Crisis Teams for Obstetric Patients

Patricia L. Dalby, MD[a],*, Gabriella Gosman, MD[b]

KEYWORDS

- Rapid response systems • Obstetric care • Crisis team • Medical emergencies

KEY POINTS

- Obstetrical care of mothers and their unborn children, involves emergencies that necessitate rapid coordination of multidisciplinary group of medical care providers efficiently. This group of providers is an obstetrical rapid response team.
- Obstetrical rapid response teams can be divided into 4 components: an afferent arm of activators, an efferent arm of responders, quality improvement personnel who track and analyze the response, and administrators that coordinate and perpetuate the efforts
- A commonly utilized training venue for obstetrical rapid response teams involves multidisciplinary simulation training. This chapter discusses simulation training and the evolution of obstetrical crisis responses over a ten year period.

Rapid response systems (RRSs) for medical emergencies, especially to avoid full cardiopulmonary arrest and facilitate trauma care, have been in existence for more than 2 decades. Continuous quality-improvement inpatient RRS teams for obstetric care involve periodic maternal and or fetal crisis situations. During events, such as fetal bradycardia, shoulder dystocia, anaphylaxis, and maternal hemorrhage, patient care needs greatly and often exceed the resources allocated to routine care. Unfortunately, these emergencies in the past decades have led to increases in maternal morbidity in the United States, especially in cases of maternal hemorrhage.[1] Many of these crises require rapid, coordinated intervention of a multidisciplinary team to optimize outcome. Increasingly, hospitals have incorporated obstetric teams into their RRSs to address these recurring but unpredictable maternal and/or fetal events. Rapid response teams focused on obstetric events differ from medical or trauma rapid response teams in that the population that they are designed to treat (pregnant women) are usually younger and healthier and the outcome of the treatment affects

Disclosure: No author has any conflicts of interest related to the content of this article.
[a] Department of Anesthesiology, University of Pittsburgh School of Medicine, Magee-Women's Hospital of UPMC, Room 3407, 300 Halket Street, Pittsburgh, PA 15213, USA; [b] Department of Obstetrics and Gynecology, University of Pittsburgh School of Medicine, Magee-Women's Hospital of UPMC, Room 3407, 300 Halket Street, Pittsburgh, PA 15213, USA
* Corresponding author.
E-mail address: dalbypl@anes.upmc.edu

Crit Care Clin 34 (2018) 221–238
https://doi.org/10.1016/j.ccc.2017.12.003
0749-0704/18/© 2017 Elsevier Inc. All rights reserved.

criticalcare.theclinics.com

2 patients (mother and fetus). Proper institution of rapid care often prevents major morbidity to both individuals.[2]

The American College of Obstetricians and Gynecologists (ACOG) Committee Opinion, "Preparing for Clinical Emergencies in Obstetrics and Gynecology," emphasizes the importance of crisis response teams for clinical emergencies relevant to obstetric patients.[3] The US Department of Health and Human Services along with the American Hospital Association and the Health Research & Educational Trust updated the Obstetrical Harm Care Change Package entitled, "2014 Update: Recognition and Prevention of Obstetrical Related Events and Harm," in which the use of obstetric RRSs were advocated.[4] Global initiatives developed recently to improve the quality of maternal and newborn care, use basic indicators of care, and advocate a coordinated obstetric care team response to emergency care. These global initiatives are based on recommendations partially spurred by the United Nations Commission on Information and Accountability for Women and Children's Health that working through the World Health Organization millennial goals program, and the Global Alliance for Surgery, Obstetric, Trauma, and Anaesthesia Care (G4 Alliance).[5,6]

Many institutions established obstetric-specific crisis teams as local quality-improvement initiatives. Recently, more reports on such teams have appeared in the published global literature.[7-13]

This article describes the implementation, training, and maintenance of an obstetric-specific crisis team at the University of Pittsburgh Medical Center (UPMC) Magee-Women's Hospital (MWH) from 2005 through 2016, including descriptions of alternate obstetric team approaches chosen by other institutions. This information was solicited through query of several medical associations (Council of Women's and Infants' Specialty Hospitals, Society for Obstetric Anesthesia and Perinatology, and Society for Simulation in Healthcare), and the Institute for Healthcare Improvement.

A current literature search of the state of art, growth and evolution, and logistics of training personnel for participation in obstetric RRS also is discussed. For many institutions, simulation training is the backbone of maintaining systemic responses and educating new providers about the RRS response. In simulation, training teams can develop a coordinated approach and communication skills required for the situations that an obstetric RRS encounter. Recent developments in simulation training specific to obstetric rapid response teams are also described. In addition, the efficacy and sustainability of obstetric RRS, with supporting data, are discussed before the conclusion of this article.

BACKGROUND AND JUSTIFICATION

The authors' institution, MWH, added an obstetric-specific team response to its RRS for multiple reasons:

1. The single call system was the most rapid way to bring multidisciplinary providers to a patient who needed care urgently. One call assembled the necessary personnel and expertise to provide optimal evaluation and intervention. After calling, the bedside provider could focus on immediate crisis care of the patient rather than making multiple sequential phone calls.
2. The multidisciplinary response facilitated interdisciplinary communication, as team responders arrived and received a briefing about the patient at nearly the same time. Poor communication was the number one root cause identified in the Joint Commission on Accreditation of Healthcare Organizations (JCAHO) Sentinel Event Alert, "Preventing Infant Death and Injury During Delivery."[14]

3. The UPMC health system had improved patient outcomes by introducing a crisis team response for inpatient prearrest medical emergencies (Condition C). After the institution of Condition C, inpatient cardiac arrests and deaths decreased.[15]
4. Incorporation of obstetric crises into the health system's RRS held promise to enhance data collection and quality efforts in obstetric care.[16]
5. The team response provided a designated team member to do real-time documentation of patient status and interventions during critical obstetric events. This promised to improve documentation problems caused by multiple providers retrospectively recording their recall of critical events.
6. Crisis response teams provided a valuable resource for staff and patient satisfaction and peace of mind. For a staff or family member who recognizes a patient in crisis, help is only a single call away.[17,18]
7. Rapid response teams have become a common response throughout the world for emergency response based on the premise that earlier intervention would produce better patient outcomes.[19]

DESIGN AND INTRODUCTION

MWH is a full-service, academic urban hospital and a tertiary referral center. It is the largest maternity hospital in Western Pennsylvania, performing more than 10,000 deliveries in 2016. At the time MWH considered adding an obstetric team, the UPMC health system already had a well-established RRS. The crisis team (Condition C) had been activated occasionally for obstetric patients. Event review of these calls suggested that the team composition was not ideal for obstetric patients. Key personnel not included on the Condition C team include obstetricians, obstetric nurses, newborn resuscitation team, and anesthesia providers. The obstetric-specific team response was called "Condition O." **Table 1** compares personnel who respond to Condition

Table 1		
Obstetric crisis versus medical crisis team responders at Magee-Women's Hospital		
	Obstetric Crisis Responders	**Medical Crisis Responders**
In-House Obstetrician	X	—
Obstetrics/gynecology resident (3rd or 4th y)	X	—
Anesthesiology MD and/or nurse anesthetist	X	—
CCM MD and CCM nurse	—	X
Patient's nurse	X	X
Administrative clinician (nurse)	X	X
L&D charge nurse	X	—
L&D clinician or manager (nurse)	X	—
Newborn resuscitation team	X	—
Respiratory	—	X
Emergency medicine MD	—	X
Resident on service	—	X
Emergency department nurse	—	X
Telemetry unit nurse	—	X
Safety/security officer	X	X

Abbreviations: L&D, labor and delivery; MD, physician; X, means providers that answer to the crisis.

O and Condition C. Some institutions have opted to use their medical crisis team to respond to obstetric patient events.

It took approximately 1 year to design and fully implement the team. The process began in early 2005 and requires constant reevaluation and revision. As the number of obstetric patients taken care of at MWH increased, so have the number of Condition O calls. Use of Condition O has been associated fewer less Condition C calls in the labor and delivery suite. **Fig. 1** shows the growth of the obstetric rapid response utilization from 2005 through 2015.

Stakeholders in the patient care areas of obstetrics, maternal-fetal medicine, obstetric nursing, critical care, neonatology, and anesthesiology convened to determine the appropriate team composition and size for the characteristics of the authors' institution. Key considerations in team composition included provision of adequate nursing manpower, involvement of anesthesia providers, involvement of newborn resuscitation providers, and capability for real-time documentation. Activation criteria for Condition O include clinical events, such as prolonged fetal heart rate decelerations, shoulder dystocia, seizure, or hemorrhage. Additionally, staff members are encouraged to call Condition O for acute situations in which a physician or nurse believes immediate evaluation/intervention is needed to avoid fetal/maternal harm. An article written in the first years of Condition O at MWH details the initial implementation and experience (trials and tribulation) of the response.[20]

Activation criteria at other institutions with obstetric teams include "staff concern" with or without a list of clinical events, such as those listed previously. Additional clinical event triggers reported by other institutions include fetal distress, prolonged fetal bradycardia, umbilical cord prolapse, absent fetal heart tones, vaginal bleeding, uterine rupture, emergent delivery, maternal respiratory distress, and maternal cardiac arrest. Some institutions have incorporated protocols that include recognition of events that can be considered triggers but not the actual onset of maternal-fetal emergencies. These triggers include, such as agitation, pain, or changes in vital signs. Such an example is that of the Modified Early Obstetric Warning System developed in Great Britain.[21]

Table 1 shows the current obstetric response team members at MWH. **Table 2** shows the roles and duties that these responders fulfill during a crisis. MWH opted for a large team with full critical care capabilities. The nursing professionals contribute the highest number of responders. This is because adequate nursing manpower is critical for implementing crisis interventions. Anesthesiology responds because they provide essential evaluation and intervention skills regarding anesthesia, analgesia,

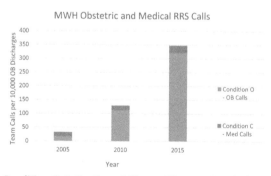

Fig. 1. Growth in Condition O Activation at Magee-Womens Hospital over time. Med, medical; OB, obstetrical.

Table 2
Obstetric crisis medical emergency team personnel and duties at Magee-Women's Hospital

Team Member		Duties
Treatment leader (obstetrician, occasionally anesthesiologist, as indicated)		Obtain briefing from appropriate person, assess team organization/composition, assess data, direct treatment, set priorities, collaborate with anesthesia team on patient plan, triage patient
Bedside nurse (usually patient's nurse)	Nursing team members select one of these roles as appropriate	Stay by patient and communicate what is going on with the condition to the patient, attach monitoring, deliver briefing to responders, report IV size/location, adjust IV rate, draw up and administer medications
Runner (L&D clinician or other personnel)		Obtain medications and equipment, deliver to appropriate person
Senior obstetric resident responder		Call for/dismiss personnel and family, call for/facilitate equipment acquisition, call for/facilitate patient transfer, get results
Nurse responder (usually L&D charge nurse)		
Documenter (usually administrative clinician)		Obtain record sheet, document (team leader, situation, vital signs and clinical data, treatments), brief personnel who come later
Procedure MD (usually ob/gyn resident)		Examine patient, inform team of maternal-fetal assessment, perform procedures
Anesthesia team (attending anesthesiologist, anesthesia residents, nurse anesthetists and student nurse anesthetists, anesthesia technicians)		Obtain briefing from obstetric team, assess analgesia, assess airway, perform anesthesia procedures, communicate anesthesia plan to team, arrange for cell salvage, collaborate with treatment leader on maternal issues
Newborn resuscitation team		Obtain briefing from obstetric team, assess newborn, resuscitate newborn

Abbreviations: IV, intravenous; L&D, labor and delivery; MD, physician; ob/gyn, obstetrics and gynecology.

airway, and hemodynamic status. A critical care medicine (CCM) physician responded in the initial 8 years of Condition O because approximately one-quarter of crises at MWH during that time were maternal crises. Later, however, responders were modified to only call CCM by a ramp-up mechanism if their services were required because of the excessive number of responders and the relative lack of CCM expertise required to resolve the emergency. Similarly respiratory therapists initially came to all Condition O responses but their services were rarely required and their presence added to the flock of responders. The neonatal resuscitation team was originally called only for gestations greater than or equal to 24 weeks. A revised policy, however, included them for every call. This change was motivated by the desire to eliminate an extra call, the need for timely arrival of the neonatal team, and gestational age uncertainty. Responders who are not needed for the crisis at hand are dismissed (ramp-down strategy). This team composition suits MWH as a high-volume, tertiary referral center with all the described providers in the hospital 24 hours a day.

Many other institutions with a high volume of obstetrics have obstetric-specific teams with personnel similar to the Condition O team. Richardson and colleagues[2] discuss the implementation and sustainability of their obstetric responses for the obstetric emergency team at Vanderbilt University; similarly, Clements and colleagues[10] discuss the obstetrical emergency response at Mary Sharp Birch Hospital in San Diego. A strategy for developing protocols for obstetric emergencies is documented using an obstetrics emergency response team and emergency drills. The protocols were drawn from sources, such as the California Maternal Quality Care Collaborative at HonorHealth Scottsdale Shea Medical Center in Scottsdale, Arizona, with successful progress in 1 protocol contributing to further protocols.[22]

In general, the obstetric rapid response teams can be divided into 4 components necessary to optimize the response within the system. These components are (1) the afferent arm that consists of activators of the response (generally the patients direct caregivers), (2) the efferent arm that consists of all the responders to call, (3) quality-improvement personnel who analyze the process, and (4) administrators who coordinate and perpetuate the effort. The following considerations may help institutions that care for smaller volumes of inpatient obstetric patients to design an appropriate obstetric team. Skills needed by a full team include (1) team leadership for data analysis and treatment decisions (this skillset may overlap with that of the team member serving in items 2, 3, and 4), (2) adult medical crisis expertise, (3) delivery/obstetric management expertise, (4) provision of anesthesia for emergency operative procedures, (5) performance of nursing tasks, (6) coordination to acquire additional resources if needed, (7) acquiring additional resources if needed, (8) newborn resuscitation, and (9) real-time documentation. **Table 3** lists potential personnel who could participate. A single individual may play multiple roles depending on the size of the team. As an alternate strategy, some institutions have opted for a ramp-up approach with a small team (1–2 individuals). This smaller team responds, rapidly assesses, and has a process to summon additional personnel with the skills listed in **Table 3** if indicated.

Staff Education

Prior to initiating Condition O, the institution held education sessions for potential callers and potential responders. Sessions occurred during staff meetings for these caregivers. Written material about Condition O appeared in institutional newsletters and as postings on patient care units. Condition O was added to the list of emergency preparedness resources on the back of employee badges. Onboarding new caregivers are now fully educated on Condition O and how to implement it.

Both callers and responders expressed initial resistance during these sessions and during the first 6 months of Condition O use. During the first few activations of the team, some physician responders criticized the caller (usually an obstetric nurse). Fear of this negative physician reaction resulted in a few Condition O calls for approximately 6 months after implementation. To overcome this, further educational efforts included case-based discussions of teamwork during critical obstetric events, review of videotaped simulated crises with Condition O versus usual sequential calling pattern, and an institutional multidisciplinary patient safety day. Facilitators of these sessions focused on 2 major points: (1) responders must not criticize the caller for summoning the team to help a patient and (2) Condition O greatly streamlines the crisis response process.

Table 3
Core skills and potential personnel to include on an obstetric team

Skill	Possible Provider Type
Team leadership	Obstetrician Critical care physician Anesthesiologist Emergency physician Hospitalist physician
Adult medical crisis expertise (airway, breathing, circulation)	Critical care physician Emergency physician Anesthesiologist Hospitalist physician CCM nurse Respiratory therapy personnel
Delivery and other obstetric management	Obstetrician Midwife Emergency physician Family medicine physician
Anesthesia for emergency procedures (or preparation for this)	Anesthesiologist Certified registered nurse anesthetist
Nursing task performance	Nurses from multiple units of the hospital (eg, obstetric care, emergency department, medical-surgical unit, ICU)
Coordination of additional resources (eg, personnel, equipment, patient transfer, crowd control)	Nurse administrator Safety/security personnel
Acquisition of additional resources (eg, medications, equipment)	Nurse Medical assistant Anesthesia technicians
Newborn resuscitation	Providers trained in newborn resuscitation (eg, obstetrician, neonatal ICU team, pediatric team, nurses)
Real-time documentation	Nurse Nurse administrator Physician

Response Team Training

Initial Condition O case review revealed opportunities for improvement in team organization, leadership, and crisis communication. In November 2005, a multidisciplinary team from MWH initiated simulation-based team off-site training at the Peter M. Winter Institute for Simulation, Education and Research. The Obstetric Crisis Team Training course trains both potential Condition O callers and responders, including obstetricians, anesthesiologists, and obstetric nurses. The course format involves online and in-person didactic presentations combined with filmed simulated emergencies and debriefing. The course curriculum was designed to meet the needs identified during the initial Condition O experience regarding team performance and specific crises encountered. Course participants learn, practice, and debrief with a focus on the following key elements: crisis communication, team organization and leadership, and appropriate emergency care.

A streamlined version of the course was also used to facilitate learning during obstetric crisis drills done in situ on MWH's patient care units. Just like in the simulation center, these drills are filmed for video-based debriefing of team performance. Many other institutions with obstetric-specific teams use simulation-based crisis team training at simulation centers and/or in situ. In situ simulation scenarios often uncover logistical or system issues unique to the specific site where they are performed and this proved true in the MWH labor and delivery suite. Structured simulation-based team training for obstetric emergencies improves patient outcomes, including hypoxic-ischemic encephalopathy, 5-minute APGAR scores less than 7, and shoulder dystocia.[23,24]

Since 2015 at MWH, monthly simulation drills of Condition O scenarios have been held in the hospital in a devoted simulation center for Condition O responders. The switch in location for the drills was made to enhance responder convenience and decrease logistical barriers to the simulation training. The focus of the training is primarily to enhance interdisciplinary communication and to build teamwork skills and relationships.

Recent Developments in Multidisciplinary Simulation Team Training for Obstetric Crisis

With the advent of the ACOG calls for RRS teams and multidisciplinary team training of these teams in 2011 and again in 2014, a proliferation of simulation training of teams has occurred and articles describing the training have been published. Several articles have recently attempted systemic review of the literature to date. One of these by Merien and colleagues[25] concluded, "Introduction of multidisciplinary team training with integrated obstetric training interventions in a simulation setting is potentially effective in the prevention of errors." They stated that studies of the overall effectiveness and the cost-effectiveness of this type of training should be undertaken, however. The TOSTI (Training Obstetrische Spoed Teams Interventie) study conducted in the Netherlands looked at the cost-effectiveness of multidisciplinary simulation-based training in obstetric emergencies. This study found the training cost effective if the sessions done in a simulation center were repeated at an actual hospital on site.[26] Later, another review of 887 articles published on the training concluded, "evidence exists for a positive impact of training in obstetric emergencies, although the majority of the available evidence applies to evaluation at the level of participants' confidence, knowledge, or skills rather than at the level of impact on clinical outcomes."[27] A study in 2009 validated the applicability of crisis team training to obstetric emergencies and found it applicable and also enhancing to the ability of the individual trainees to accurately assess their own performances.[28]

Several articles focused on teamwork education itself, and 1 made recommendations about this type of training and the context in which the program was delivered in, the diversity of the teams itself, and the tools used in the education programs.[29,30] It is the authors' opinion that these articles should be essential background reading for anyone contemplating developing a teamwork education program. Another article found that multidisciplinary team simulation training in an obstetric model could translate to improved teamwork in other settings.[31]

A Dutch group has looked at the impact of multiprofessional simulation-based team training on many aspects of health care (discussed previously).[26] They also studied, however, the effect of such training on patient-reported quality of care, finding improved patient perceptions of obstetric care 6 weeks postpartum when measured by the Pregnancy and Childbirth Questionnaire.[32] They also investigated the effect of team training on team performance and medical technical skills and found improvements in both areas.[33]

Another emphasis in the field has been on the development of valid teamwork assessment tools that can be used both for simulation training and for quality assessment of actual events. Several groups have done extensive work in this regard and have developed tools that may be used to evaluate the effectiveness of an obstetric rapid response team for ongoing quality assurance. The Canadian group along with some American colleagues developed the Perinatal Emergency Team Response Assessment (PETRA) scale that they validated using high-fidelity simulation scenarios. They found this scale, which had a 5-point rating scale for shared mental model, communication, situational awareness, leadership, followership, and workload management as well as an overall score, valid and reliable.[34] Prior to publishing this data Balki and colleagues[35] (also of the PETRA scale investigation) had performed along with others a meta-analysis using the preexisting publications concerning teamwork assessment tools developed for obstetric emergencies. In this meta-analysis, they found 3 scales the most reliable; the Clinical Teamwork Scale, the Global Assessment of Obstetric Team Performance, and the Global Rating Scale of performance. The meta-analysis concluded, however, that all 3 scales were lacking in some aspects of validity and quality.[35]

Data Collection, Review, and Process Improvement

The hospital developed a peer review process of the obstetric crisis team calls, which was similar to the review of cardiac arrests and medical crisis team calls. Obstetric crisis event records and patient medical records are reviewed by a designated physician to detect opportunities to improve patient management, team function, or systems issues that may have resulted in or influenced the crisis. Details of each team response are entered into the hospital's code response database. Multiple improvements have resulted from issues identified in obstetric crisis team events and crisis team drills. Additional major patient safety interventions that have resulted from this event review include interdisciplinary rounds every 4 hours on the labor and delivery unit and an increased number of attending obstetricians supervising care on the unit 24 hours a day. In addition, a special group of hospitalist obstetricians was also developed, who expressly work in the obstetric triage unit and the labor and delivery suite at MWH.

With the UPMC system-wide implementation of the electronic medical record (EMR), the written Condition O record was adopted to the EMR system. The advantage of the electronic Condition O record is that the timing of the events and the patients' vital signs are documented in real time in conjunction with the electronic recording of the fetal heart rate. The EMR version of the Condition O record was also introduced in the simulator training.

Institutions initiating an obstetric-specific crisis response might consider collecting data on the following: (1) event rate; (2) event location; (3) reason for the call; (4) services provided by the team; (5) time (and duration) of initial call, team arrival, and end of resuscitation; (6) maternal and fetal clinical characteristics; (7) maternal and fetal/neonatal clinical outcomes; and (8) patient events for which the team should have been called but was not. Staff perception of the patient safety environment in obstetric care services may also give valuable feedback about the obstetric crisis team.

The following patient outcome measures may help assess the impact of an obstetric crisis team. For events with emergency concerns about fetal well-being that result in cesarean section (prolonged bradycardia, cord prolapse, and so forth), collect data on time from decision for cesarean section to incision (decision to incision), APGAR scores, cord blood gases, and unanticipated neonatal ICU admission. For patients with obstetric hemorrhage, collect data on the number and type of blood products administered, estimated blood loss, and unanticipated hysterectomy. For shoulder dystocia events, collect data on the time from delivery of the newborn's head to delivery of the body (head-to-body interval), APGAR scores, cord blood gases, and neonatal fracture and nerve injuries. Timely and regular debriefing after such incidents reinforces the safety environment. Data on the performance of debriefing and timeliness to the particular incident may be fruitful.

National Initiatives for Rapid Response Teams

As part of a national initiative, led by the Institute for Healthcare Improvement, there was a how-to guide generated from data of 5 million incidents of medical harm between 2006 and 2008. This can serve as a basic guide to any group contemplating setting up such a response to obstetric emergencies with in their maternal-fetal/neonatal care facility. It contains numerous suggestions on which data to gather, how to analyze the data, and general quality investigation and assurance.[30]

USAGE OF CONDITION O AT MAGEE-WOMEN'S HOSPITAL AND DISCUSSION

Providers began using Condition O regularly beginning approximately 6 months after its introduction. **Fig. 1** shows crisis team call rates for obstetric patients 2005 to 2016. **Table 4** shows the reasons a caregiver activated a Condition O response and the maternal, fetal, and combined maternal fetal indications that occurred at MWH. **Box 1** indicates reasons for calling a maternal medical RRS in a MWH labor and delivery suite, but these were often called as Condition O because caregivers were more used to making the Condition O call. **Box 1** shows the reasons for Condition O calls

Table 4		
Indications for obstetric crisis team activation, June 2005 through December 2013, listed in decreasing frequency of occurrence for each category		
	Indication	**Number of Events**
Fetal	Nonreassuring fetal heart rate (prolonged deceleration, heart rate lost, and so forth)	Most frequent
	Shoulder dystocia	
	Cord prolapse	
	Imminent or precipitous delivery term	
	Imminent or precipitous delivery preterm	
	Imminent delivery of fetus with malpresentation (footling breech, face, and so forth)	
	Difficult delivery during cesarean section	
	Preterm labor	
	Rupture of membranes off of the obstetric unit	
	Contraction/abdominal/back pain off the obstetric unit	
	Head entrapment during breech delivery	Least frequent
Maternal	Postpartum hemorrhage	Most frequent
	Seizure	
	Syncope or lightheadedness	
	Patient unresponsive	
	Postpartum hypoglycemia	
	Respiratory distress	
	Chest pain/pressure	
	Possible intravenous injection of epidural medications	
	Upper gastrointestinal bleeding	Least frequent
Both	Abruption	Most frequent
	Antepartum vaginal bleeding	
	Hemorrhaging placenta previa	
	Home delivery preterm	Least frequent

Box1
Indications for medical crisis team activation for obstetric patients, June 2005 through January 2013 (listed in decreasing order of events)

Most frequent
   Syncope or lightheadedness
   Seizure
   Postpartum hemorrhage
   Respiratory distress
   Hemorrhage due to miscarriage
   Patient unresponsive
   Change in mental status
   Trauma or fall
   Anaphylaxis
   Hypotension
   Chest pain

Least frequent

---

and indicates their relative frequency. Providers called Condition O primarily for threats to fetal well-being; fetal well-being indication for a Condition O call has increased up to 90% in the recent years. Use of the team for this indication suggests that the single call mechanism allows caregivers (especially nursing) to focus on patient care interventions instead of summoning each member of the team individually. Emergencies that pose a direct risk to both mother and fetus made up 10% of calls. Pure maternal crises constituted the other percentage of events. Obstetric caregivers are now instructed to call Condition C for reasons that are purely maternal indications. During education sessions for on-boarding staff and in MWH simulation training sessions instructions are given for staff that an initial call can always be upgraded to a more serious condition. An example of this is that an initial call by a caregiver of a condition O situation could be upgraded to a Condition A if the maternal situation worsens to a cardiac or pulmonary arrest.

Most Condition O calls come for patients on in the labor and delivery suite and the obstetric triage unit. These units are adjacent to each other and staffed with multiple obstetricians, anesthesia personnel, and multitiered nursing providers. During the initial 6 months of Condition O, many nurses and physicians highlighted the ready availability of personnel on the unit. For this reason, they did not perceive that an obstetric crisis response team was needed. Routine staffing on the unit, however, is targeted to routine patient needs. Condition O use patterns demonstrate that providers' attitudes have shifted to recognize the periodic need for a rapid bolus of care resources. **Table 5** shows the patient locations for Condition O and calls on obstetric patients and their relative frequency.

Condition O patient events divert patient care resources from lower-acuity to higher-acuity patients. This has raised the concern that the crisis response abandons lower-acuity patients. Condition O events thus far, however, have not resulted in staffing shortages for other obstetric patients at MWH. The median duration of Condition O responses is less than 10 minutes. A majority of team members disband after a brief event review. Remaining members document the event for the medical record (physician team leader, several minutes) and for code response data collection (nurse administrator, 5–30 minutes). Further review of the condition response occurs at the every 4-hour patient safety interdisciplinary meetings that occur on the labor and delivery suite but rarely elicit long discussion. The event if complicated is discussed later at multidisciplinary quality-improvement conferences that occur quarterly at MWH.

Table 5
Obstetric crisis team activation locations, June 2010 through June 2013

Location	Number of Events/Year
Labor and delivery	>100
Triage unit	>40
Antepartum unit	>20
Emergency department	>20
Postpartum unit	>20
Ultrasound department	<10
Parking lot	<5
Cafeteria	<5
Staff meeting room	<5
Obstetric clinic	<5

Providers initially expressed concern that the Condition O response would scare patients and families. Unsolicited patient comments at the authors' institution, however, indicate that patients and family are not frightened by the sudden influx of personnel and flurry of activity during Condition O. This feedback suggests that patients and their families perceive the crisis team response as evidence of high-quality emergency care. An anonymous quality-improvement survey project at MWH of patients and families who had experienced a Condition O queried their reactions to the event. The surveys found that both parties believed they had appreciated the prompt and organized response to their emergency. Also, the survey was validated and proved a reliable tool as a patient and family satisfaction questionnaire that can be used for obstetric emergency situations (see **Table 6**) (Zhan J, Kwon C, Stein K, et al. Patient and family satisfaction following emergency obstetric crisis: development of a valid and reliable questionnaire. Abstract: at Society for Obstetrical Anesthesiology and Perinatology [SOAP] 2014 annual meeting proceedings, unpublished).[36]

A need for patient and family education about what a Condition O response is, what occurs during the response, and the possibility of a Condition O call during their hospitalization was identified at MWH. Some institutions, including the authors', have rapid response team information on their Web site. Also many, including MWH, have rapid response team literature and/or posters that they use to educate patients and families on the chance they may experience such an event during their hospital stay.

Table 6
Patient and family satisfaction tool for obstetric emergency response

Questionnaire	Family	Patient
Cronbach α	0.841	0.905
Test-retest Pearson R	0.85	0.80
Subscale correlation	0.806	0.850

The patient and family satisfaction questionnaire in obstetric crisis has been found psychometrically sound with regards to measurement of satisfaction with care and medical decision making of patients and families. The questionnaire contains 2 different subscales—the first segment, which is composed of 10 items, focuses on satisfaction with overall care, and the second, which is composed of 2 Likert items and 3 comment free-writing sections, assesses satisfaction regarding medical decision making. All questions used Likert-5 response scales.

Providers have used Condition O at a steady rate at the authors' institution. An obstetric-specific RRS team may be particularly important for institutions with lower-volume and/or lower-acuity obstetric units. Such units have fewer staff present 24/7 and fewer crises. For such institutions, a designated team may facilitate efficient training of team members and an improved response to obstetric crises.

Continuous Quality Improvement and Evaluation of Obstetric Rapid Response Systems

In 2014, the entire Condition O response at MWH was reevaluated with the goal of optimization of the process from both provider and patient perspectives. The most recent two years of Condition O data were reviewed and discussed. Five areas of concern were identified with the MWH Condition O response at that time and recommendations generated as follows.

Area of concern 1: definition of the optimal response team and the training of the team members
At this reevaluation period, the analysis of the MWH Condition O history revealed that an overwhelming majority of conditions were called for perceived need of immediate delivery, for actual delivery problems (ie, shoulder dystocia), or for immediate post-partum problems. At this time, the needs for routine CCM (ICU staff) and respiratory therapy staff were found not required for the efferent arm of the response. Neonatal ICU team members remained an integral part of the response on labor and delivery Condition O calls but were no longer required to respond to calls to the postanesthesia care unit or postpartum units. A new hospital-based multidisciplinary simulation training course was developed after this reorganization that emphasized the new team and team communication and interactions.

Area of concern 2: determination of the leadership of the Condition O response and the delineation of the roles of the various team responders
With review of the preceding 10 years of Condition O responses, it became obvious that an obstetrician (usually a hospitalist general obstetrician) had been the primary leader of the responses. Thus, the leadership was designated to the labor suite generalist obstetrician unless a patient's primary obstetrician desired to maintain leadership or there was a reason for other leadership because of the situation (ie, anesthesiologists became the leaders if the patient was having an anaphylactic attack). One of the perceived problems with the Condition O response was that there were an overwhelming number of responders and there was a need to ramp down the response. At the time of the analysis, it was determined that the senior obstetric resident rotating in the labor and delivery room was the best person to do this because of knowledge of which responders would be required for a particular Condition O call. This resident was also charged with coordinating in conjunction with the labor and delivery nursing supervisor on duty the resources and locations to be used for the response. The patient's primary nurse was charged with staying with the patient and communicating the response to the patient and family who might become alarmed by the group of responders entering their situation in haste. The other roles of the responders did not require any change, especially in light of improved real-time documentation of the response with the designated documenter using an EMR format.

Area of concern 3: further evaluation of the triggers for a Condition O call and elimination of barriers for the calling of a Condition O response
Recent criticism at the time of the reevaluation of called Condition O events by certain providers (primarily supervisory caregivers) had resulted in adverse psychological

impact on potential future calls of Condition O responses (primarily the patients' direct caregivers.) This represented a serious backsliding of the original intent of the Condition O response. Broad all-party agreement and reinforcement of the concept that nurses and any other obstetric patient caregiver could initiate a Condition O response changed the behavior of the parties that had been critical. This validated the already established criteria to trigger a Condition O and the concept that any clinical deterioration would be grounds for making the call.

Area of concern 4: establishment of an optimal debriefing process for Condition O responses and a schedule of Condition O group meetings to assure continuous quality improvement

Consensus was reached that all condition O responses would be debriefed after the event at the every 4-hour interdisciplinary group safety rounds, held in a common area in the labor and delivery suite. A mechanism was developed to feed the Condition O information forward to the labor and delivery charge nurse of the specifics of the response to be discussed at the rounds if the particular responders could not be present at the 4-hour period.

Area of concern 5: establishment of robust mechanisms for patient education prior to the occurrence of a Condition O

A need for additional patient information about the possibility of a condition and what would happen was identified. This was accomplished by adding additional information to computerized electronic records, patients' consents, and the obstetric Web site. New posters and direct signage in the patient's rooms were introduced. All patient caregivers were instructed to debrief the patients and their familie about a Condition O possibility and to debrief them after a response as soon as clinically possible.

These 5 areas of concern are issues that were identified as having become problematic with the MWH initial Condition O response and prompted the restudy of the response. It is likely that these 5 areas of concern are similar to issues that might develop with any large health care center's obstetric emergency RRS. These areas of concern may need to be reviewed periodically (along with other concerns that may be identified) on a periodic basis to ensure the sustainability of an obstetric specific rapid response team.

Efficacy and Sustainability of Obstetric Multidisciplinary Rapid Response Systems

Patient safety initiatives are commonly criticized because of the inability to detect and demonstrate a causal link between process change and outcome. Obstetric quality and patient safety indicators are in need of evaluation and revision to boost their ability to discriminate between high-quality and low-quality care.[2,37] This revision process is currently under way. Future measures may improve the ability to evaluate the impact of patient safety initiatives, such as Condition O. In the modern patient safety environment, however, clinical areas often have multiple safety and quality-improvement projects ongoing at any given time. Thus, it can be difficult to show a causal link between a specific initiative and a specific patient outcome measure.

Part of the justification for introduction of Condition O was to apply a health system's successful experience with the RRS to a different clinical setting, widely recognized as high risk and in need of periodic emergent multidisciplinary expert care. Condition O accomplished the goal of providing a reliable and effective resource that improves the patient care process. It is a resource that hospital staff members have used with consistent frequency since 2006. This provides evidence of both staff satisfaction with the process and a safety culture change.

At MWH, Condition O has not had a detectable impact on the perinatal quality and safety data collected and reported by the authors' institution. These parameters include The Joint Commission Obstetrical Pregnancy and Related Conditions Core Measures, the Agency for Healthcare Research and Quality Perinatal Patient Safety Indicators, the National Perinatal Information Service/Quality Analytic Services Obstetric Quality Indicators, and the Adverse Outcome Index. Specifically, these include event rates of vaginal birth after cesarean section, third-degree or fourth-degree laceration, obstetric trauma, postpartum readmissions, wound complications, anesthesia complications, neonatal mortality, birth trauma injury to neonates, and birth trauma linked to maternal shoulder dystocia, The Adverse Outcome Index includes maternal deaths, intrapartum neonatal death, uterine rupture, unplanned maternal ICU admission, birth trauma, return to the operating room or labor and delivery, neonatal ICU admission greater than or equal to 37 weeks and greater than or equal to 2500 g, maternal blood transfusion, and third-degree or fourth-degree laceration. Many of these measures are not directly related to the crisis team activities. Some of the potentially relevant outcomes, such as maternal and neonatal death, are such rare events that crisis team impact is difficult to assess.

The institution also evaluated malpractice claims data for possible impact of Condition O on malpractice activity. Not enough time has elapsed, however, since 2005 to assess the impact on professional liability activity, given the long statute of limitations on obstetric cases.

Recent publications have indicated that obstetric emergency teams may have begun to translate into tangible medical improvements and patient outcomes. One article from South Korea indicated that many obstetric emergencies were treated successfully on the general wards and there was a reduction of the number of ICU admissions for critically ill obstetric patients.[12] Improvements in the outcomes of major obstetric hemorrhage have occurred coincident with the implementation an obstetric response team in conjunction with other team responses for care of the bleeding obstetric patient.[38,39] Rapid response mechanisms using mobile technology have improved obstetric outcomes in areas lacking prior resources.[13] Decreases in cesarean delivery team decision to incision times have come with the implementation of obstetric rapid response teams, although not necessarily with better neonatal outcomes.[40] Ascension Health system adapted an RRS approach to shoulder dystocia within more than 40 hospitals with positive results.[41] An individual patient's primary team used for rapid response systemic care has been shown to reduce unexpected hospital mortality.[42]

Sustained RRSs for any sort of patient care are time and labor intensive, and the actual positive results tend to be difficult to measure in patient care. The idea of rapid notification of patient deterioration and a systemic response to it, however, seem logical. There have been some literature suggestions that may improve the sustainability of such a response.[19,42] The critical care nursing profession has had some of the best simple suggestions on sustainable practices.[43] The plan-do-study-act method of systemic evaluation also has been used successfully to improve obstetric rapid response teams.[44]

SUMMARY

An obstetric-specific crisis team allows institutions to optimize the care response for patients with emergent maternal and/or fetal needs. Characteristics of an optimal obstetric rapid response team are team member role designations; streamlined communication; prompt access to resources; and ongoing education, rehearsal, and training along with continual team quality analysis. The outcomes of the team quality analysis then must be incorporated into future team responses and reinforced in training. The team response provides a key resource to reassure staff, physicians, and patients that prompt crisis care is only a single call away. Data on the obstetric-specific crisis response at MWH show that team activation is common, improves the care process, and has promise to improve outcomes directly and/or through event analysis and subsequent process improvement.

REFERENCES

1. Callaghan WM, Creanga AA, Kuklina EV. Severe maternal morbidity among delivery and postpartum hospitalizations in the United States. Obstet Gynecol 2012; 120:1029–36.
2. Richardson MG, Domardradzki KA, McWeeney DT. Implementing and obstetrical emergency team response system: overcoming barriers and sustaining dose response. Jt Comm J Qual Patient Saf 2015;41(11):514–21.
3. American College of Obstetricians and Gynecologists Committee on Patient Safety and Quality Improvement. ACOG committee opinion no. 590: preparing for clinical emergencies in obstetrics and gynecology. Obstet Gynecol 2014; 123(3):722–5.
4. Obstetrical Harm Care Change Package 2014 Update; recognition and prevention of obstetrical related events and harm. Available at: www.hret-hen.org/index.php. Accessed September 11, 2017.
5. Madaj B, Smith H, Mathai M, et al. Developing global indicators for quality of maternal and newborn care: a feasibility assessment. Bull World Health Organ 2017;95:445–452l.
6. Haider A, Scott JW, Gause CD, et al. Development of a unifying target and consensus indicators for global surgical systems strengthening: proposed by the global alliance for surgery obstetric, trauma, and anaesthesia care (The G4 Alliance). World J Surg 2017. https://doi.org/10.1007/s00268-017-4028-1.
7. Guise JM. Anticipating and responding to obstetric emergencies. Best Pract Res Clin Obstet Gynaecol 2007;21(4):625–38.
8. Al Kadri HM. Obstetric medical emergency teams are a step forward in maternal safety! J Emerg Trauma Shock 2010;3(4):331–415.
9. Clark ES, Fisher J, Arafeh J, et al. Team training/simulation. Clin Obstet Gynecol 2010;53(1):265–77.
10. Clements CJ, Flohr-Rincon S, Bombard AT, et al. OB team stat: rapid response to obstetrical emergencies. Nurs Womens Health 2007;11:194–9.
11. Crozier TM, Galt P, Wilson SJ, et al. Rapid response team calls to obstetrical patients in a busy quaternary maternal hospital. Aust N Z J Obstet Gynaecol 2017. [Epub ahead of print].
12. Baek MS, Son J, Huh JW, et al. Medical emergency team may reduce obstetric intensive care unit admissions. J Obstet Gynaecol Res 2017;43(1):106–13.
13. Davila-Torres J, Gonzalez-Izquirdo J, Ruiz-Rosas RA, et al. Rapic response obstetrics team at insituto mexicano del seguro social, enabling factors. Cir Cir 2015;83(6):492–5.
14. Joint Commission on Accreditation of Healthcare Organizations (JCAHO). Preventing infant death and injury during delivery. Sentinel Event Alert 2004;30:1–3.
15. DeVita MA, Braithwaite RS, Mahidhara R, et al. Use of medical emergency team responses to reduce hospital cardiopulmonary arrests. Qual Saf Health Care 2004;13(4):251–4.

16. Braithwaite RS, DeVita MA, Mahidhara R, et al, Medical Emergency Response Improvement Team (MERIT). Use of medical emergency team (MET) to detect medical errors. Qual Saf Health Care 2004;13(4):255–9.
17. Galhotra S, Scholle CC, Dew MA, et al. Medical emergency teams: a strategy for improving patient care and nursing work environments. J Adv Nurs 2006;55(2): 180–7.
18. PSNet (Patient Safety Network) Rapid Response Systems/AHRQ Patient Safety Network. Available at: https://psnet.ahrq.gov/primers/primer/4/rapid-response-systems. Accessed September 1, 2017.
19. Jones DA, DeVita MA, Bellomo R. Rapid response teams (current concepts). N Engl J Med 2011;365(2):139–46.
20. Gosman GG, Baldiseri M, Stein K, et al. Introduction of an obstetric-specific medical emergency team for obstetric crises: implementation and experience. Am J Obstet Gynecol 2008;198(4):367.e1-7.
21. Singh S, McGlennan A, England A, et al. A validation study of the CEMACH recommended modified early obstetric warning system (MEOWS). Anaesthesia 2012;67:12–8.
22. Roth CK, Parfitt SE, Hering SL, et al. Developing protocols for obstetric emergencies. Nurs Womens Health 2014;18(5):379–90.
23. Draycott T, Sibanda T, Owen L, et al. Does training in obstetric emergencies improve neonatal outcome? BJOG 2006;113(2):177–82.
24. Draycott TJ, Crofts JF, Ash JP, et al. Improving neonatal outcome through practical shoulder dystocia training. Obstet Gynecol 2008;112(1):14–20.
25. Merien AER, Van de Ven J, Mol BW, et al. Multidisciplinary team training in a simulation setting for acute obstetric emergencies. Obstet Gynecol 2010;115: 1021–31.
26. Van de Ven J, Van Baaren GJ, Fransen AF, et al. Cost-effectiveness of simulation-based team training in obstetric emergencies (TOSTI study). Eur J Obstet Gynecol Reprod Biol 2017;216:130–7.
27. Calvert KL, Mcgurgan PM, Debenham EM, et al. Emergency obstetric simulation training: how do we know where we are going, if we don't know where we have been? Aust N Z J Obstet Gynaecol 2013;53:509–16.
28. Robertson B, Schumacher L, Gosman G, et al. Simulation-based crisis team training for multidisciplinary obstetric providers. Simul Healthc 2009;4(2):77–83.
29. Eddy K, Jordan Z. Stephenson M Health professionals' experience of teamwork education in acute hospitals settings: a systemic review of qualitative literature. JBI Database System Rev Implement Rep 2016;14(4):96–137.
30. 5 million lives campaign. Getting started kit: rapid response teams. Cambridge (MA): Institure for Healthcare Improvement; 2008. Available at: www.ihi.org.
31. Van der Nelson HA, Siassakos D, Bennett J, et al. Multiprofessional team simulation training, based on an obstetric model can improve teamwork in other areas of health care. Am J Med Qual 2014;29(1):78–82.
32. Truijens SE, Banga FR, Fransen AF, et al. The effect of multiprofessional simulation-based obstetric team training on patient-reported quality of care: a pilot study. Simul Healthc 2015;10(4):210–6.
33. Fransen AF, Van de Ven J, Merien AER, et al. Effect of obstetric team training on team performance and medical technical skills: a randomized controlled trial. BJOG 2012;119(11):1387–93.
34. Balki M, Hoppe D, Monks D, et al. The PETRA (Perinatal Emergency Team Response Assessment) scale: a high-fidelity simulation validation study. J Obstet Gynaecol Can 2017;39(7):523–33.e12.

35. Onwochei DN, Halpern S, Balki M. Teamwork assessment tools in obstetric emergencies (a systemic review). Simul Healthc 2017;12(3):165–76.
36. Wall RJ. Refinement, scoring, and validation of the family satisfaction in the intensive care unit (FS-ICU) survey. Crit Care Med 2007;35(1):271–9.
37. Grobman WA. Patient safety in obstetrics and gynecology: the call to arms. Obstet Gynecol 2006;108(5):1058–9.
38. Skupski DW, Brady D, Lowenwirt IP, et al. Improvement in outcomes of major obstetric hemorrhage through systemic change. Obstet Gynecol 2017;130(4):770–7.
39. Gillespie C, Sangi-Haghpeykar H, Munnur U, et al. The effectiveness of a multidisciplinary, team-based approach to cesarean hysterectomy in modern obstetric practice. Int J Gynaecol Obstet 2017;137(1):57–62.
40. Wacks MA, Andrew M, Nelson K, et al. Effect of rapid response cesarean delivery team decision-to-incision time on fetal outcome. Obstet Gynecol 2015 [abstract: 05001]. Available at: http://journals.lww.com/greenjournal/Abstract/2015/05001/Effect_of_Rapid_Response_Cesarean_Delivery_Team.175.aspx.
41. Burstein PD, Zalenski DM, Edwards JL, et al. Changing labor and delivery practice: focus on achieving practice and documentation standardization with the goal of improving neonatal outcomes. Health Serv Res 2016;51(6 part II):2472–86.
42. Howell MD, Ngo L, Folcarelli P, et al. Sustained effectiveness of a primary-team-based rapid response system. Crit Care Med 2012;40(9):2562–8.
43. Lazzara EH, Benishek LE, Sonesh SC, et al. The 6 "Ws" of rapid response systems; best practices for improving development, implementation, and evaluation. Crit Care Nurs Q 2014;37(2):207–18.
44. Smith K, Leash J, Cadawas T, et al. Abstract: improving obstetric rapid response teams: multidisciplinary simulation training utilizing the Plan-Do-Study-Act cycle. Proceedings of the 2013 AWHONN convention. J Obstet Gynecol Neonatal Nurs 2013;42:S56.

A Decade of Difficult Airway Response Team

Lessons Learned from a Hospital-Wide Difficult Airway Response Team Program

Lynette Mark, MD[a,b,]*, Laeben Lester, MD[c,d],
Renee Cover, BSN, RN, CPHRM[e], Kurt Herzer, MD, PhD[f]

KEYWORDS

- Difficult airway response team • Rapid response teams • Difficult airway patient
- Multidisciplinary airway management • Simulation-based medical education
- Hospital difficult airway alert systems • Difficult airway registry • Second victim

KEY POINTS

- Difficult airway adverse events continue to be the fourth most common event in the American Society of Anesthesiologists closed claims database, with devastating consequences to patients, families, providers, and institutions.
- Multidisciplinary airway teams have been shown to reduce emergency surgical airways and the associated morbidity and mortality.
- The Johns Hopkins Hospital Difficult Airway Response Team (DART) program has integrated operations, safety, and educational components designed to improve multidisciplinary teamwork and communications, reduce airway-related adverse events, and promote innovative educational activities for airway providers.
- Institutions interested in initiating a DART program can use the Johns Hopkins program as a roadmap for developing a similar initiative.

[a] Department of Anesthesiology and Critical Care Medicine, Johns Hopkins Medicine Multidisciplinary Airway Programs, Difficult Airway Response Team (DART) Program, Johns Hopkins Medicine, 1800 Orleans Street, Baltimore, MD 21287, USA; [b] Department of Otolaryngology–Head and Neck Surgery, Johns Hopkins Medicine Multidisciplinary Airway Programs, Difficult Airway Response Team (DART) Program, Johns Hopkins Medicine, 1800 Orleans Street, Baltimore, MD 21287, USA; [c] Department of Anesthesiology and Critical Care Medicine, Johns Hopkins Medicine Multidisciplinary Airway Programs, Johns Hopkins Medicine, 1800 Orleans Street, Baltimore, MD 21287, USA; [d] Department of Emergency Medicine, Johns Hopkins Medicine Multidisciplinary Airway Programs, Johns Hopkins Medicine, 1800 Orleans Street, Baltimore, MD 21287, USA; [e] Johns Hopkins Health System Legal Department, The Johns Hopkins Hospital, 1800 Orleans Street, Baltimore, MD 21287, USA; [f] Oscar Health, 219 Withers Street, Brooklyn, NY 11211, USA
* Corresponding author. Johns Hopkins Medicine, 1800 Orleans Street, ZB 6214, Baltimore, MD 21287-8711.
E-mail address: lmark@jhmi.edu

Crit Care Clin 34 (2018) 239–251
https://doi.org/10.1016/j.ccc.2017.12.008
0749-0704/18/© 2018 Elsevier Inc. All rights reserved.

criticalcare.theclinics.com

INTRODUCTION

Difficult airway adverse events continue to be the fourth most common type of adverse event in the American Society of Anesthesiologists (ASA) closed claims database, with devastating consequences to patients, families, providers, and institutions.[1] Patients with difficult airways present unique challenges in emergency situations, particularly outside the operating room, increasing the risk of life-threatening complications, including anoxic brain injury, death, and long-term disability. In the ASA closed claims analysis, respiratory-related events were twice as likely in remote locations than in the operating room (OR).[2] Litigation related to these events may result in significant settlement costs, including structured settlements for those patients with permanent neurologic disability, often resulting from anoxic brain injury. Although the events are likely underreported and national data on prevalence are not currently collected, the state of Maryland lists airway events resulting in death and disability as the sixth most common reported adverse event, after falls, pressure ulcers, surgical events, delays in treatment, and medication errors, but the second highest fatality rate of all events.[3]

A decade ago (2008-2018) the Johns Hopkins Hospital Difficult Airway Response Team (DART) program was created as a multidisciplinary effort to prevent airway-related morbidity and mortality after evaluating a series of actual or near miss events related to emergency difficult airway management between 2005 and 2007. Root cause analysis indicated that a major factor in airway event morbidity and mortality was the lack of a systematic approach for responding to difficult airway patients in an emergency. Common themes across these adverse events were inconsistent paging/communication, lack of availability of advanced and specialized airway equipment, insufficient training/experience of providers for advanced and specialized procedures, lack of a mechanism for reliably enlisting more experienced physicians, and unclear definition of roles and responsibilities during a multidisciplinary airway event. In addition, the authors made the following observations:

- All events occurred outside the OR environment.
- Four primary disciplines were involved anesthesiology and critical care medicine (ACCM), otolaryngology–head and neck surgery (OHNS), trauma surgery (TS), and emergency medicine (EM)
- Although each discipline had recognized difficult airway experts—at national and international levels—the authors had not effectively leveraged their expertise to form a coordinated, multidisciplinary approach to complex airway management at the institution.

A business plan was drafted to fund the startup and operational costs of what would become the DART program. An oversight committee was formed to lead the DART program, which included physician representation from ACCM, OHNS, TS, and EM as well as risk managers, safety officers, human factors engineers, and Lean Six Sigma experts.

DIFFICULT AIRWAY RESPONSE TEAM PROGRAM: GOALS AND DESIGN

The DART program had 5 goals:

1. Establish a coordinated, multidisciplinary emergency response process for managing adult difficult airway patients.
2. Decrease the risk of adverse airway events resulting in permanent disability or death.

3. Minimize institutional liability related to adverse airway events.
4. Improve provider communication and education.
5. Disseminate information about difficult airway management to patients and other providers.

The structure of the DART program was built around 3 pillars, and new processes were developed within each:

1. Operations and quality improvement. The focus was on simplification of activating multiple specialty DART providers by using the emergency paging system's "universal" phone number that activates code and emergency rapid response teams. Code team activations could be escalated to DART if requested by any bedside provider during a patient event. DART activation results in attending physicians from ACCM, OHNS, and TS coming to the bedside within 10 minutes or less. Based on review of DART activations, standardized DART carts were developed and strategically placed throughout the institution to facilitate delivery of specialty equipment to the bedside when a DART call is activated. Respiratory therapists are trained to assist with the DART cart setup and use. On arrival to the bedside, a brief DART time-out is performed to ensure agreement on the airway management plan and roles. Every DART event is entered into a confidential internal airway registry for subsequent review by the DART oversight committee. Equipment specialists process all DART carts within 3 hours, and units are notified of the locations of backup DART carts in the event of another DART activation. See **Fig. 1** for an example of a DART cart. Patients are provided with educational materials to ensure future continuity of care.
2. Safety. In the first year of the DART program's existence, in situ simulations of difficult airway events were conducted in 5 different hospital units with high-fidelity simulators to evaluate and mitigate system defects. A multitude of defects were identified that resulted in systems improvements, including improved method of team paging and activation, elevator key placement on all DART carts, refinement

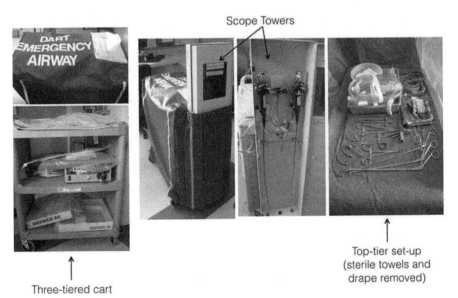

Scope Towers

Top-tier set-up
(sterile towels and
drape removed)

Three-tiered cart

Fig. 1. DART cart. This photograph shows the organization of a standard DART cart.

of DART cart supplies (eg, safety scalpels instead of nonretractable scalpels and scope hanging case), assignment of DART parking space at the emergency room entrance, and development of a DART cart inventory and safety checklist. Quarterly multidisciplinary DART case review conferences were also held for continuous learning and process improvement.

3. Education. A DART program multidisciplinary difficult airway course was developed by DART practitioners and presented quarterly for senior house staff and airway support staff to standardize training across departments and teach advanced airway management techniques through lectures and simulations. Web-based DART education learning modules were also created for all staff members. Policies and procedures were created and then updated and approved by the medical board every 3 years. Multidisciplinary institutional grand rounds for DART are held biannually. Joint faculty appointments were initiated for DART faculty departmental leaders to foster multidisciplinary teamwork, communications, training, and academic advancement.

DIFFICULT AIRWAY RESPONSE TEAM PROGRAM: RESULTS

In 2015, the authors published a comprehensive article on the DART program that provided an overview of DART program implementation, analysis of DART airway event data, inventory lists for DART carts, cost considerations for DART operations, in situ simulation results, and a DART program implementation package to assist other institutions in developing a DART program.[4]

Between 2008 and 2013, there were 4738 code activations that were escalated to a DART 360 times (7.5%); 29 (8%) of these required emergency surgical airways, and 62 (17.2%) of patients were stabilized and transported to the OR for definitive airway management in a controlled environment. Risk factors for DART activation included body mass index greater than 30, history of difficult airway, history of head and neck tumor, history of chronic obstructive pulmonary disease, history of tracheostomy, current tracheostomy, limited cervical spine range of motion, airway edema (nonallergic), angioedema, and active airway bleeding (**Box 1**). Direct laryngoscopy, fiberoptic bronchoscopy, and videolaryngoscopy (VL) were the most frequent techniques used. The use of rigid laryngoscopy by OHNS reduced the need for surgical airways in many cases, improving patient outcomes. Standardization of emergent surgical cricothyroidotomy techniques resulted in no adverse patient complications when performed. See **Fig. 2** for the program's 5-step approach.

Box 1
Risk factors for Difficult Airway Response Team patients

Body mass index >30

History of difficult airway

History of head and neck tumor

History of cervical spine injury

History of angioedema

Current tracheotomy

History of chronic obstructive pulmonary disease

Current airway bleeding

Previous tracheotomy

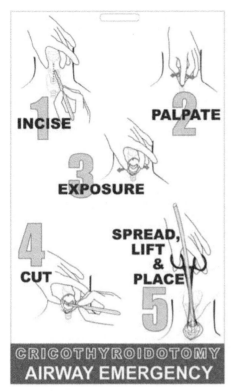

CALL 5-4444

Tell Operator:
1. "I need the difficult airway response team!"
2. Building Name, Floor, Room #, Unit Phone #

AIRWAY CART LOCATIONS:

Area	Location	Phone
ED	Trauma Bay (G1332)	5-2280
NCCU	3005B Alcove	5-8070
ZBOR	Next to Room 315	5-8075
PICU	Across from Room 19	5-5260
CVSICU	Across from Room 15	5-4826
L & D	Outside OR 1	5-5850
SICU	Across from Room 53	5-5370
MICU	10180A Alcove	5-5570
Wbg OR	Room 3333	2-1223
WICU	Nurse Manager Office	2-1048
Wbg 5	Between B & C (5261)	5-8880
JHOC	PACU (Room LL055)	5-4006
MPCU	Main Nurses Station	5-5340
Hal 2	Alcove H268	7-3127

WHO WILL ARRIVE:
ACCM Attending/Senior Resident
Trauma Attending & Senior Resident
OLHN Attending (in house 7a-5p and on-call 5p-7a)
OLHN Senior Resident (in house)
Respiratory Therapy

Fig. 2. DART airway emergency card. An example of a laminated card all DART providers receive detailing the steps for performing an emergency cricothyroidotomy and for DART activation and DART cart locations.

During this time, 18 DART multidisciplinary difficult airway courses were taught, resulting in the training of more than 200 providers; 20 ACCM grand rounds problem-based learning DART cases were presented; and 5 institutional DART program multidisciplinary grand rounds were presented.

Overall, there were no airway-related deaths, sentinel events, or malpractice claims for adult patients managed by DART during this first 5-year period. At the 10-year mark, the DART program continues to sustain these results—there have been no airway-related deaths, sentinel events, or malpractice claims for adult patients.

LESSONS LEARNED

1. Clarify attending roles when you arrive at the bedside: "Who's in charge?"

   When a DART is activated and members arrive at the patient bedside, there is an immediate briefing and formulation of an airway plan, backup plans, optimal location (bedside, unit, or OR) and responsibilities of each individual. Once a primary plan is agreed on, attending physicians work together to optimize patient care.

   The authors clarified attending roles to prevent confusion or disagreement at an actual event:

   - ACCM attending: pharmacology, physiology, mask ventilation, noninvasive airway techniques (eg, mask airway, supraglottic devices, VL, fiberoptic

intubation and bronchoscopy, and emergent surgical cricothyroidotomy in the event that an airway needs to be immediately established prior to the arrival of OHNS, TS, or EM attending present)
- OHNS attending: noninvasive airway techniques (eg, fiberoptic intubation and bronchoscopy, rigid laryngoscopy, and bronchoscopy) and emergent surgical cricothyroidotomy[5]
- TS attending: noninvasive airway techniques (bronchoscopy) and emergent surgical cricothyroidotomy
- EM attending: pharmacology, physiology, mask ventilation, noninvasive airway techniques and emergent surgical cricothyroidotomy

2. Agree on a standardized approach for airway management for all specialties.

To avoid disagreements between different disciplines regarding preferred algorithms or guidelines for airway management, it is important that a standardized approach for airway management be agreed on by all involved DART program specialties. For example, ACCM members adhere to the ASA guidelines (**Fig. 3**),[6] but the other specialties have their own professional practice standards, with preferred alternative approaches. Collaboration to optimize utilization of the different specialty approaches enhances care and treatment of patients.

To address this, the authors combined the ASA difficult airway guidelines with the Vortex approach, introduced by Chrimes (**Fig. 4**).[7,8] The Vortex approach facilitates graphic visualization of the progression from noninvasive airway techniques, such as face mask ventilation, placement of supraglottic airway (SGA), or endotracheal tube, advising no more than 3 attempts per each—to a standardized surgical technique if noninvasive techniques are unsuccessful. Incorporation of the Vortex approach into operations, safety, and educational programs has resulted in a more comprehensive understanding and consistent application of airway management decisions at DART events by all DART providers.

3. Maintain fiberoptic intubation and bronchoscopy skills, because they remain the gold standard for awake intubation and select asleep airway management scenarios.

Despite emerging airway technologies that have replaced many instances in which awake fiberoptic intubation was the airway technique of choice in some instances, patients presenting with complex physiology and pathology may benefit from awake techniques. In the program's institution, awake fiberoptic intubation remains the technique of choice in cases of angioedema, select head and neck pathology (eg, major resections with abnormal pathology and/or very limited mouth opening, sublingual tumors), patients who have had failed supraglottic device mask ventilation, and select cases of significant morbid obesity (**Box 2**, Case 1).

4. Remember that a surgical airway is not a failed airway and might be the optimal choice.

Pre-DART review of emergency airway events indicated that a proactive, standardized, awake/open tracheostomy or urgent/emergency cricothyroidotomy, performed by attending physicians in OHNS and TS (or with direct supervision of senior house staff), can be the primary airway management technique of choice for select DART events. A laminated airway emergency card was created that all DART providers received (see **Fig. 2**). Standardization of emergency surgical airway techniques resulted in no adverse patient complications when performed. In the first 5 years of DART, 6 surgical

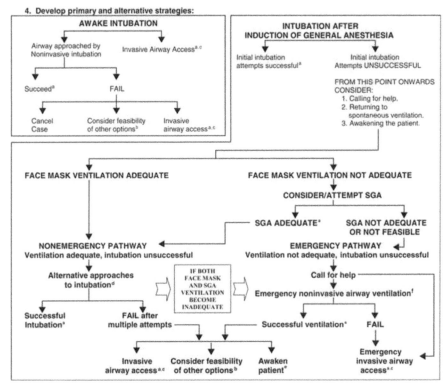

Fig. 3. ASA difficult airway algorithm, 2013. [a] Confirm ventilation, tracheal intubation, or SGA placement with exhaled CO_2. [b] Other options include (but are not limited to) surgery using face mask or SGA anesthesia (eg, LMA, ILMA, and laryngeal tube), local anesthesia infiltration, or regional nerve blockade. Pursuit of these options usually implies that mask ventilation will not be problematic. Therefore, these options may be of limited value if this step in the algorithm has been reached via the emergency pathway. [c] Invasive airway access includes surgical or percutaneous airway, jet ventilation, and retrograde intubation. [d] Alternative difficult intubation approaches include (but are not limited to) video-assisted laryngoscopy, alternative laryngoscope blades, SGA (eg, LMA or ILMA) as an intubation conduit (with or without fiberoptic guidance), fiberoptic intubation, intubating stylet or tube changer, light want, and blind oral or nasal intubation. [e] Consider repreparation of the patient for awake intubation or canceling surgery. [f] Emergency noninvasive airway ventilation consists of an SGA. (*From* Apfelbaum JL, Hagberg CA, Caplan RA, et al. Practice guidelines for management of the difficult airway: an updated report by the American Society of Anesthesiologists Task Force on Management of the Difficult Airway. Anesthesiology 2013;118(2):251–70; with permission.)

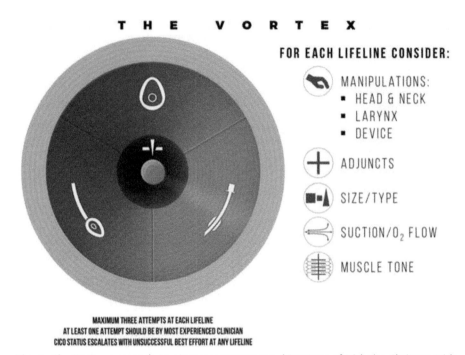

Fig. 4. The Vortex approach to airway management. (*Courtesy of* Nicholas Chrimes; with permission.)

airways were averaged per year without morbidity or mortality. Preliminary review of data from DART years 6 to 10 demonstrates a similar experience (see **Box 2**, Case 2).

5. Keep pace with advances in airway management innovations.

For process improvement of the quarterly DART program airway course, 2 airway management innovations were identified that have since been incorporated into the curriculum: ORSIM bronchoscopy simulator (Airway Simulation Limited, Auckland, New Zealand)[9,10] and Difficult Airway Algorithm and Rescue Cricothyrotomy (DAARC) Web-based program.[11]

The ORSIM can simulate oral and nasopharyngeal, laryngeal, tracheal, and bronchial pathology to simulate difficult upper and lower airway problems. Physically the model consists of a replica flexible bronchoscope, a digital sensor, and a computer. The bronchoscope is inserted into the digital sensor and the computer creates virtual scenarios, visible on the screen that replicates a real-world bronchoscope monitor.

DAARC was created to standardize the Veterans Health Administration team approach to non-OR airways and reduce adverse outcomes from surgical airways. The DAARC educational systems consist of video didactics, podcasts, and an innovative training program that relies on serious gaming in place of traditional live simulation for complex and dynamic clinical decision making. Simulation outcomes include the use of the cognitive aid (Vortex), time to obtain a successful airway, number of attempts in each technique, number of attempts with an optimization of each technique, time interval from failure of nonsurgical interventions until cricothyrotomy, and time from recognition of need surgical rescue to front of neck access.

Box 2
Difficult Airway Response Team case examples

Case 1: A 50-year-old woman presented to an emergency department with angiotensin-converting enzyme inhibitor–induced angioedema, with onset over the past 3 hours to 4 hours. On physical examination, she had significant lip and tongue edema and a reported change in phonation. She had no stridor or respiratory distress and arterial oxygen saturation (Sao_2) was 98% on room air. A DART was activated. OHNS performed a nasopharyngoscopy and noted supraglottic edema (Chiu category classification type 3).[25] The patient was transferred to the OR for airway management. In the OR, in a sitting position, she was nasally topicalized by ACCM while OHNS prepped and topicalized her neck, including a transtracheal lidocaine. A nasal trumpet with endotracheal adaptor was inserted into her right nares to provide supplemental oxygen and verify ventilation while an endotracheal tube was inserted into her left nares for the fiberoptic bronchoscope. There was significant supraglottic and glottic swelling and the intubation was challenging. Tracheal intubation was verified with continuous waveform capnography and the patient was sedated and transferred to the medical ICU for further care.

Case 2: A 49-year-old male patient, postoperative day 2 from a large ventral hernia repair was extubated without incident. Several hours later, he experienced respiratory distress, and the decision was made to reintubate him. ACCM was called and reviewed the OR record, which identified airway management with easy mask ventilation and intubation with VL with an angulated blade. The patient was induced with propofol and rocuronium and noted to be a difficult mask airway. VL with an angulated blade failed to reveal the glottic opening and a supraglottic device was attempted without success. A DART was activated. A nasal and oral airway were placed with evidence of some ventilation and maintenance of Sao_2 88% to 90%. On arrival, OHNS and TS attending physicians worked together and quickly established an emergency cricothyroidotomy, with their standardized technique and a vertical skin incision. The patient had no neurologic complications or adverse complications from the surgical airway and was successfully decannulated a few days later.

Case 3: A 65-year-old patient, body mass index of 60, presented to the emergency department with hypoxic, hypercapnic respiratory failure. He was transferred to the MICU for management and became increasingly obtunded, not responding to continuous positive airway pressure. ACCM was called for urgent intubation. On examination, he was a Mallampati grade 4 with large tongue, full beard, and unknown intubation history. A DART was activated. He was ramped and preoxygenated for 10 minutes with both nasal cannula 15 L and bag-valve-mask with the ZOLL R series continuous waveform capnography. With Sao_2 98%, the patient was induced with propofol and succinylcholine. Laryngoscopy with the McGrath X blade failed to visualize the glottic opening secondary to extensive redundant tissue. The OHNS attending visualized the glottic opening with the Holinger rigid laryngoscopy, advanced an Eschmann stylet and subglottic endotracheal tube successfully, and verified placement with continuous waveform capnography and bilateral breath sounds. Sao_2 was maintained between 98% and 96% for the entire procedure.

---

6. Collect and use data to continually improve.

Every DART event is reviewed by the DART oversight team for quality of care delivered including successful and unsuccessful airway management techniques. Examples of items removed from the DART cart because of issues with emergency use include percutaneous cricothyroidotomy kits, jet ventilation, and nonsafety scalpels. Likewise, VL was successful when used in the OR but had less success with DART use at the bedside. Although VL is not a technique currently on the DART cart, many ICUs acquired them, making VL readily available at DART activations. The authors identified, however, that the institution had 3 different VL brands and that not all ICUs had purchased the angulated/difficult airway blade. This was rectified and VL has become a highly successful DART technique.

Another process improvement includes a change in practice to ensure verification of oxygenation and ventilation during DART events. To minimize hypoxia during airway manipulation and ensure effective ventilation, continuous waveform capnography is used during all of aspects of airway management, including mask ventilation, verification of endotracheal intubation/successful surgical airway, and immediate post–airway management and transport. The authors initiated an institutional best practices standard of providing high-flow nasal oxygenation at 15 L/min via nasal cannula, in addition to bag-valve-mask preoxygenation, during airway management and are currently exploring other oxygenation techniques that can deliver up to 30 L per minute nasally during airway management.[12,13] The program's institution upgraded automated external defibrillators to the ZOLL R series (ZOLL, Chelmsford, MA),[14] which facilitates continuous waveform capnography, and initiated best practices, such that all aspects of airway management are verified by continuous waveform capnography—the same gold standard used for all patients receiving any form of anesthetic/airway management in the program's ORs, surgical ICUs, and remote locations[15] (see **Box 2**, Case 3).

As the institution expanded, the authors worked with human factors engineers and safety officers to expand the number of DART carts and mapped out coverage for each ward or ICU to ensure a 10-minute delivery metric. The DART cart locations are displayed on the back of the cricothyroidotomy airway emergence badge (see **Fig. 2**) given to DART team members, with a more comprehensive list/backup DART cart chart available in each patient care area.

7. Create a pediatric DART program

When the DART program was initiated in 2008, there were numerous discussions regarding emergency difficult airway management care for pediatric patients and the establishment of a pediatric DART (pDART) program. The decision was made to develop an adult DART program that would provide coverage to all pediatric patients—specifically to assist in initial assessment and stabilization while pediatric specialists could be mobilized.

From 2008 to 2015, the DART program was activated for 30 pediatric patients, with 90% of these in non-OR locations; 50% of these patients were stabilized by DART and transferred to an OR for definitive airway management by pediatric specialists. Primary successful airway techniques were direct laryngoscopy (30%), OHNS laryngoscope (23%), fiberoptic bronchoscope (14%), VL (12%), and SGA (2%); 7 (12%) surgical airways were performed.

Despite best efforts by the adult DART program and pediatric specialists, the authors realized that the pediatric population had unique challenges, prompting a re-evaluation of creation of a separate pDART program. A formal pDART program business plan was submitted to the institution and was funded. The pDART program emulates the adult DART program's 3 core components and additionally customizes difficult airway management to pediatric patients with a comprehensive consultation service focusing on preventative measures to ensure an airway management plan is in place, particularly for children with craniofacial anomalies.

8. Do not forget the second victim: the aftermath of adverse airway events for providers.

The aftermath of adverse airway events can lead to many victims: the first victims are the patient and family/friends, the second victim is the health care provider involved in the event, and the third victim is the institution at large.[16,17] During the program's pre-DART event review, many practitioners were emotionally traumatized. The authors built into the DART program extensive support initiatives that included 24-hour review by an oversight team with direct communication to DART members, referrals to a faculty staff and assistance program, peer-to-peer support, and multidisciplinary grand rounds with supportive discussions. In 2011, the institution formalized the Resilience in Stressful Events Team (RISE) program[18] and collaborated with the DART program to include more physicians/airway experts in the RISE program, attend rise peer responder basic and advanced seminars, and participate in the Maryland Patient Safety Center resilience training seminar.[19] Institutions interested in addressing second victims are encouraged to access additional comprehensive materials available on the Web.[20–23] See **Box 3** for a summary of lessons learned.

DISCUSSION

Institutions considering developing a rapid response team focused on difficult airway management can learn from the experience of the Johns Hopkins Hospital DART program. The decision to implement a full DART program, similar in scope to what is described in this article, likely depends on existing expertise for airway management, human and financial resources, and the unique patient populations served by the institution in question. To help facilitate the dissemination of the DART program, the authors have developed an implementation package that includes numerous tools, templates of policies and procedures, and other resources to assist interested institutions.[4]

In 2015, the University of Rochester Medical Center (URMC) adapted and implemented the Johns Hopkins Hospital DART Program at the URMC Strong Memorial Hospital, demonstrating the feasibility of adaptation.[24] This initiative was sponsored by MCIC Vermont, a medical malpractice insurance company, through the Risk Reduction Awards Program.

The Johns Hopkins Hospital DART program oversight committee reviewed the URMC-MCIC proposal and provided guidance in adapting the Johns Hopkins Hospital DART program to align with the unique issues and resources at URMC. The URMC principal investigator participated in a Johns Hopkins on-site review of the DART program and had access to DART tool box resources (**Table 1**), with ongoing monthly consultation. URMC implemented the DART program within 3 months and is currently

---

Box 3
Lessons learned from the Difficult Airway Response Team program

1. Clarify attending roles when you arrive at the bedside: "Who's in charge?"

2. Agree on a standardized approach for airway management for all specialties.

3. Maintain fiberoptic intubation and bronchoscopy skills, because they remain the gold standard for awake intubation and select asleep airway management scenario.

4. Remember that a surgical airway is not a failed airway and might be the optimal choice.

5. Keep pace with advances in airway management innovations.

6. Collect and use data to continually improve.

7. Create a pDART program.

8. Do not forget the second victim: the aftermath of adverse airway events for providers.

Table 1
Johns Hopkins Hospital interdisciplinary clinical practice manual for patient care: Difficult Airway Response Team adult policy

Table of Contents	Page Number
I. OBJECTIVES	1
II. INDICATIONS FOR USE	1
III. DEFINITIONS	2
IV. RESPONSIBILITY	2
V. PROCEDURE	4
VI. REPORTABLE CONDITIONS	6
VII. DOCUMENTATION	7
VIII. EDUCATION AND COMMUNICATION	7
IX. SUPPORTIVE INFORMATION	8
X. SIGNATURES	8
Appendix A: Difficult Airway Wrist Band	
Appendix B: DART Cart Audit	
Appendix C: Bedside Difficult Airway Alert Card	
Appendix D: Patient Education	
Appendix E: DART Cart Daily Equipment Checklist	
Appendix F: Emergency Paging Phone Card	
Appendix G: DART Cart Locations	
Appendix H: DART Cart Backup Plan	
Appendix I: Elevator Access	
Appendix J: Bronchoscope Cleaning Sign	
Appendix K: Medic Alert Foundation Difficult Airway/Intubation Registry	

Keywords: airway, airway cart, airway equipment, D.A.R.T., DART, difficult airway, emergency.

in their third year of practice, with reported 49 successful DART activations. The URMC experience demonstrates that the DART program can be implemented at other institutions with fidelity to the original design.

In conclusion, implementation of the Johns Hopkins Hospital DART program has led to improved patient outcomes, standardized and advanced airway management curricula, fostering multidisciplinary teamwork, and decreased institutional liability.

REFERENCES

1. Metzner J, Posner KL, Lam MS, et al. Closed claims analysis. Best Pract Res Clin Anaesthesiol 2011;25:263–76.

2. Metzner J, Posner KL, Domino KB. The risk and safety of anesthesia at remote locations: the US closed claims analysis. Curr Opin Anaesthesiol 2009;22(4): 502–8.

3. Office of Health Care Quality. Maryland Hospital patient safety program fiscal year 2015 annual report. Catonsville (MD): Maryland Department of Health & Mental Hygiene; 2015.

4. Mark LJ, Herzer KR, Cover R, et al. Difficult airway response team: a novel quality improvement program for managing hospital-wide airway emergencies. Anesth Analg 2015;121(1):127–39.

5. Hillel AT, Pandian V, Mark LJ, et al. A novel role for otolaryngologists in the multi-disciplinary difficult airway response team. Laryngoscope 2015;125(3):640–4.
6. Apfelbaum JL, Hagberg CA, Caplan RA, et al. Practice guidelines for management of the difficult airway. Anesthesiology 2013;118(2):251–70.
7. Chrimes N. The vortex: a universal "high-acuity implementation tool" for emergency airway management. Br J Anaesth 2016;117:i20–7.
8. Chrimes N, Fritz P. The vortex approach to airway management. Available at: http://vortexapproach.org. Accessed October 30, 2017.
9. Baker PA, Weller JM, Baker MJ, et al. Evaluating the ORSIM simulator for assessment of anesthesists' skills in flexible bronchoscopy: aspects of validity and reliability. Br J Anaesth 2016;117:i87–91.
10. Baker PA. ORSIM. Available at: www.orsim.co.nz. Accessed October 30, 2017.
11. Feinleib J. DAARCGame. Available at: www.sharedfedtraining.org/external_content/DAARCweb/DAARC/index.html. Accessed October 30, 2017.
12. Weingart SD, Levitan RM. Preoxygenation and prevention of desaturation during emergency airway management. Ann Emerg Med 2012;59(3):165–75.
13. Patel A, Nouraei SA. Transnasal humidified rapid-insufflation ventilator exchange (THRIVE): a physiological method of increasing apnoea time in patients with difficult airways. Anaesthesia 2015;70(3):323–9.
14. Zoll R. Series monitor defibrillator. Available at: www.zoll.com/medical-products/defibrilattors/r-series. Accessed October 30, 2017.
15. Whitaker DR. Time for capnography - everywhere. Anaesthesia 2011;66:541–9.
16. Wu AW. Medical error: the second victim. The doctor who makes the mistake needs help too. BMJ 2000;320(7237):726–7.
17. Seys D, Wu AW, Gerven EV, et al. Health care professionals as second victims after adverse events: a systematic review. Eval Health Prof 2012;36(2):135–62.
18. Johns Hopkins Medicine RISE Program: resilience in stressful events team. Available at: www.safeathopkins.org/resources/johns-hopkins/rise/index.html. Accessed October 30, 2017.
19. Sexton B. Enhancing caregiver resilience essentials. Available at: www.dukepatientsafetycenter.com. Accessed October 30, 2017.
20. Medically Induced Trauma Support Services. Available at: www.mitss.org. Accessed October 30, 2017.
21. Missouri University Health Center forYOU Team. Available at: www.muhealth.org/about/quality-of-care/office-of-clinical-effectiveness/foryou-team/. Accessed October 30, 2017.
22. Joffe AM. Use your SMARTs (some kind of multidisciplinary airway response team) for emergent airway management outside the operating room. Anesth Analg 2015;121:11–3.
23. Chmielewska M, Winters BD, Pandian V, et al. Integration of a difficult airway response team into a hospital emergency response system. Anesthesiol Clin 2015;33:369–79.
24. Borovcanin Z, Shapiro J, Oren H, et al. Difficult Airway Response Team (DART) Program at University of Rochester Medical Center: adaption of the Johns Hopkins Medicine DART Program to improve patient outcomes. World airway management meeting. Dublin, Ireland. 2015.
25. Chiu AG, Newkirk KA, Davidson BJ, et al. Angiotensin-converting enzyme inhibitor-induced angioedema: a multicenter review and an algorithm for airway management. Ann Otol Rhinol Laryngol 2010;119(12):836–41.

Sepsis Rapid Response Teams

Tammy Ju, MD[a,1], Mustafa Al-Mashat, MD[b,1],
Lisbi Rivas, MD[a,1], Babak Sarani, MD[a,*]

KEYWORDS

- Septic shock • Sepsis • Infection

KEY POINTS

- Sepsis rapid response teams can improve patient outcomes.
- Protocol-based therapies in the treatment of septic shock have been shown effective.
- Hospital-wide quality-improvement initiatives are the backbone of the rapid response team.

BACKGROUND

Sepsis remains the leading cause of death in critically ill patients. Septic shock continues to carry a mortality risk of 20% to 40%, contributing to approximately 1 in every 3 deaths in the United States.[1,2] Studies have shown that the best predictors of improved mortality outcome are early recognition of septic shock and timely administration of antibiotics.[3,4] Rapid response teams (RRTs) provide an ideal means to achieve these goals for hospitalized patients outside the ICU.

Sepsis is defined as a syndrome of dysregulated host response to infection leading to life-threatening organ dysfunction.[5,6] Unlike other life-threatening conditions, like acute coronary events, stroke, or trauma, early sepsis syndrome can be initially associated with subtle nonspecific signs that are easy to miss. Additionally, numerous previous clinical trials attempting to target key factors that are inappropriately elaborated or not cleared, such as nitric oxide or lipopolysaccharide, have not demonstrated mortality benefit.[7] Rather, some have found increased mortality. Thus, the standard of care remains early recognition of septic shock and implementation of a treatment bundle centered on optimizing perfusion, obtaining source control when possible, and delivery of appropriately dosed, broad-spectrum antibiotics within 1 hour of onset of shock.[8]

Disclosures: The authors do not have any financial or commercial interests to disclose.
[a] Department of Surgery, George Washington University, 2150 Pennsylvania Avenue, NW 6B, Washington, DC 20037, USA; [b] Department of Internal Medicine, George Washington University, 2150 Pennsylvania Avenue, NW 6B, Washington, DC 20037, USA
[1] Present address: c/o Dr Babak Sarani, 2150 Pennsylvania Avenue, NW 6B, Washington, DC 20037.
* Corresponding author. 2150 Pennsylvania Avenue, NW 6B, Washington, DC 20037.
E-mail address: bsarani@mfa.gwu.edu

As in many life-threatening conditions, early identification of sepsis is key. Identification of septic patients and the implementation of early resuscitation along with early antibiotic administration seem to be what makes the difference in these patients' outcomes; hence, early goal-directed therapy is recommended by the Surviving Sepsis Campaign.[3,8] This strategy focuses on early resuscitation with fluids and pressors (when needed) and the early administration of antibiotics when a bacterial infection is suspected, while monitoring for end-organ ischemia as a guide for ongoing resuscitation. Multiple barriers have been identified, however, when it comes to the management of septic patients: these include the inability to continuously monitor all hospitalized patients, the inability to recognize critical illness early on, and the inability to use available resources when needed.[3] Aside from providing resources for timeliness of resuscitation and antibiotic therapy, RRTs and medical emergency teams (METs) provide clinicians who are versed in the latest resuscitation methods and treatment modalities for septic shock. In net sum, a sepsis RRT can provide the needed multidisciplinary expertise and resources to implement the evidence-based guidelines put forth by various national organizations as best practice for the initial management of septic shock.

SEPSIS RAPID RESPONSE TEAMS: WHAT ARE THEY? HOW ARE THEY DIFFERENT FROM OTHER RAPID RESPONSE TEAMS?

One important resource available to address the initial evaluation and timely initiation of treatment to critically ill patients is an RRT/MET dedicated and trained specifically to manage septic patients in a standardized fashion. Health care systems have started to incorporate sepsis as a specific entity when it comes to activating the rapid response system (RRS), with the main goal of raising awareness among health care providers and staff on the importance of early identification and early management of these patients. These teams are typically multidisciplinary, consisting of nurses, respiratory therapists, critical care staff, and pharmacists who are trained in recognition and implementation of sepsis-specific protocols.

The dedicated sepsis RRT/MET evaluates these patients in a standardized fashion, using established diagnostic criteria, such as systemic inflammatory response syndrome (SIRS)/sequential organ dysfunction assessment (SOFA) scores, modified early warning scores (MEWS), or basic physiologic and laboratory work parameters to identify at-risk patients. Patients who are hypotensive (systolic blood pressure <90 mmHg, or mean arterial pressure <60 mmHg) or normotensive, with concerning signs of tachypnea, skin mottling, acute encephalopathy, oliguria, or lactic acidosis, benefit from having a dedicated team that follows a standardized treatment protocol.[9]

What makes sepsis response teams different is their education in early sepsis recognition, resuscitative therapy, and rapid administration of appropriate antibiotic treatment, often as part of a hospital-wide initiative. To augment the ability to administer antibiotics in a timely fashion, large hospitals can include a clinical pharmacist as part of the responding team.[10] This sepsis RRT, which is specifically educated in sepsis management, can then choose the ideal antibiotics based on an antibiotic algorithm specific to the hospital.[11] This forward planning has been shown to improve both the timely administration of antibiotics as well as the probability of appropriately covering the offending microbe(s).

OUTCOMES AFTER IMPLEMENTATION OF SEPSIS RAPID RESPONSE TEAM/MEDICAL EMERGENCY TEAM

The concept of an RRS was described in the 1990s.[12,13] Since then, the implementation of an RRS has been shown to significantly reduce time to intensivist arrival, time to fluid administration, and time to ICU admission. Studies have also specifically explored the effect of these response teams in the nontraumatic shock population with similar results and, most importantly, with decreased overall patient mortality.[9,14] Sebat and colleagues[14] performed a single-center prospective study over 7 years from 1998 to 2005, which showed that education of frontline providers, protocol goal-directed therapy, RRT activation, intensivist involvement, and ICU mobilization decreased time to treatment and resulted in a sustained decrease in hospital-wide sepsis-related mortality. A study published in 2004 examined the use of MET at a university hospital setting in postoperative patients who showed any sign of physiologic instability and demonstrated that the introduction of an ICU-based MET decreased mortality rate and mean hospital stay.[15] A retrospective study in 2016 showed that delays in RRT activation are independently associated with worse patient morbidity and mortality outcomes.[16]

Recent studies, in particular one by the Surviving Sepsis Campaign published in 2015, have also shown that increased compliance with "protocol-based therapy bundle" is associated with a 25% relative risk reduction in in-hospital mortality.[17] Another important study elucidating the effects of protocol-based bundle therapies is the Michigan Health & Hospital Association Keystone Sepsis Collaborative project published in 2016, which showed that high bundle adherence hospitals had significantly greater improvements in sepsis-related hospital mortality and hospital length of stay compared with those hospitals who had low adherence.[18] This study found that hospitals that implemented a protocol-based resuscitation bundle for management of septic shock had a 2% to 3% absolute reduction in in-hospital mortality and a 1-day reduction in length of stay over a 4-year period. This study used a concurrent control group of hospitals to separate out secular trends in outcomes, thereby estimating the independent effect of the collaborative.

Yet some randomized control trials exploring this protocol-based effect have not shown any additional benefit compared with the standard of care.[19] So what makes the difference? Specific to the Keystone Sepsis Collaborative is a detailed explanation of the cultural improvement component and education of such bundles that is likely what makes the difference. Although the Keystone study did not show improved outcomes in septic shock patients beyond current trends, the key is the high bundle adherence related to quality-improvement initiatives, leadership support, and increasing receptiveness to changing methodology, which likely contribute to overall improved outcomes.[18] Thompson and colleagues[18] describe these strategies starting with collaborative multidisciplinary teams provided with educational toolkits about sepsis, education on up-to-date evidence-based treatment of those in septic shock, and clinical tools for standardization of care. Additionally, face-to face-workshops with consistent re-education and coaching as part of the continued quality-improvement protocol-based intervention are key to maintain competency and lasting outcomes.

A recent study published in the *Journal of Critical Care* in 2017 based in Jacksonville, Florida, using a retrospective chart review investigated the effect of a sepsis alert program on patient outcomes.[20] At this large regional referral center, it was found that a hospital-wide program using electronic recognition and RRT intervention improved outcomes in patients with sepsis. Specifically, they reported a significant reduction in mortality, need for mechanical ventilation, length of ICU stay, and overall hospital stay, which also translated into a significant reduction in hospital charges. Again, a large hospital-wide education initiative was developed and implemented, targeted at both bedside providers and the RRT itself. Specifically described in this initiative was not only an automated sepsis screening in the electronic health record but also an RRT nurse proactively seeking out high-risk patients on the general wards. Furthermore, an automated "possible sepsis notification" in the electronic health record using the MEWS–sepsis recognition score (SRS) was used to identify patients at risk. Once patients were identified, a sepsis alert was called, which included an order set for laboratory tests, antibiotic recommendations (institution specific), initial fluid bolus, and blood cultures. It also paged providers, including physicians and nurses directly, and allowed a sepsis protocol bundle to be administered. A pharmacist also had the ability to review each patient's microbiologic history for further tailored therapy. The investigators described the goal of this study as to instill a "culture change regarding sepsis care throughout our institution," which they hypothesized was largely due to education, the use of the electronic recognition of high-risk patients, sepsis alert order bundle, and RRTs for specific areas of the hospital.[20]

THE USE OF CLINICAL ASSESSMENT TOOLS

There are various scoring systems that seek to identify patients with probable sepsis early on in their hospital course. The single most sensitive sign of sepsis, however, is tachypnea. Tachypnea is an early sign of both critical illness and sepsis, although it lacks specificity for any single cause.

There have been multiple clinical assessment criteria described to aid in identifying septic patients outside of the ICU. Most recently, the Quick SOFA (qSOFA) score has been recommended for use as a prompt to consider possible sepsis.[21] Rather than the use of the less specific SIRS, qSOFA is meant to be sepsis specific, focused, and easy to use. The qSOFA score, however, as with any other predictive system, has not been prospectively validated in non-ICU patients with presumed or possible sepsis. Another useful tool to use for early identification of septic patients is the MEWS.[22] Guirgis and colleagues[20] described a modified MEWS-SRS protocol with a positive predictive value of 70% for sepsis. Both the qSOFA and MEWS-SRS scores use the respiratory rate as an important point to trigger further evaluation in hospitalized patients.

With the advances of the electronic medical records, alerts can be generated automatically to increase awareness of the possibility of sepsis or critical illness and help in the decision to activate the RRS.[20] These objective criteria can be integrated into the sepsis RRT and may be useful in early recognition of a potentially deteriorating patient. This premise, however, has yet to be validated prospectively.

BARRIERS IN HEALTH CARE

Culture change is one of the biggest barriers preventing implementation of better practices. Following a standardized protocol in the management of septic patients has the potential to improve patient outcomes but depends on the degree of adherence to the protocol implemented within the hospital.[18] Providing ongoing education to staff can be beneficial, and assuring the availability of a specialized team (sepsis RRT) can likely lead to improved outcomes due to defined roles of the team members, assuring the competency of the team.[14] But this is easier said than done. Despite the availability of an RRS and ongoing encouragement to activate it when the clinical picture is concerning, evidence suggests that there frequently are delays in the process, leading to worse outcomes.[3] The many reasons that account for this are discussed elsewhere but are equally applicable to the care of the septic patient. Ultimately, resources; consistency by which providers are educated and, more importantly, reeducated on better system practices; and up-to-date evidence on how to treat and manage septic patients are recurrent themes found among successful implementation of the sepsis RRS.[14,15,20] Whereas hemodynamic monitoring and electronic medical records constitute a small portion of the overall solution to the challenge of identifying and appropriately treating septic patients early, it is the expectation that sepsis RRSs will be used regularly and staffed and resourced appropriately to mitigate unnecessary morbidity and mortality.

REFERENCES

1. Angus DC, Linde-Zwirble WT, Lidicker J, et al. Epidemiology of severe sepsis in the United States: analysis of incidence, outcome, and associated costs of care. Crit Care Med 2001;29(7):1303–10.
2. Liu V, Escobar GJ, Greene JD, et al. Hospital deaths in patients with sepsis from 2 independent cohorts. JAMA 2014;312(1):90–2.
3. Kumar A, Roberts D, Wood KE, et al. Duration of hypotension before initiation of effective antimicrobial therapy is the critical determinant of survival in human septic shock. Crit Care Med 2006;34(6):1589–96.
4. Rivers E, Nguyen B, Havstad S, et al. Early goal-directed therapy in the treatment of severe sepsis and septic shock. N Engl J Med 2001;345:1368–77.
5. Singer M, Deutschman CS, Seymour CW, et al. The Third International Consensus definitions for sepsis and septic shock (sepsis-3). JAMA 2016;315:801–10.
6. Shankar-Hari M, Phillips GS, Levy ML, et al, Sepsis Definitions Task Force. Developing a new definition and assessing new clinical criteria for septic shock: for the Third International Consensus definitions for sepsis and septic shock (sepsis-3). JAMA 2016;315:775–87.
7. Vincent JL, Abraham E. The last 100 years of sepsis. Am J Respir Crit Care Med 2006;173:256–63.
8. Rhodes A, Evans LE, Alhazzani W, et al. Surviving sepsis campaign: international guidelines for management of sepsis and septic shock: 2016. Intensive Care Med 2017;43(3):304–77.
9. Sebat F, Johnson D, Musthafa AA, et al. A multidisciplinary community hospital program for early and rapid resuscitation of shock in nontrauma patients. Chest 2005;127(5):1729–43.
10. Sarani B, Brenner SR, Gabel B, et al. Improving sepsis care through systems change: the impact of a medical emergency team. Jt Comm J Qual Patient Saf 2008;34(3):179–82, 125.
11. Miano TA, Powell E, Schweickert WD, et al. Effect of an antibiotic algorithm on the adequacy of empiric antibiotic therapy given by a medical emergency team. J Crit Care 2012;27(1):45–50.
12. Lee A, Bishop G, Hillman KM, et al. The medical emergency team. Anaesth Intensive Care 1995;23(2):183–6.
13. Bristow PJ, Hillman KM, Chey T, et al. Rates of in-hospital arrests, deaths and intensive care admissions: the effect of a medical emergency team. Med J Aust 2000;173(5):236–40.
14. Sebat F, Musthafa AA, Johnson D, et al. Effect of a rapid response system for patients in shock on time to treatment and mortality during 5 years. Crit Care Med 2007;35(11):2568–75.
15. Bellomo R, Goldsmith D, Uchino S, et al. Prospective controlled trial of effect of medical emergency team on postoperative morbidity and mortality rates. Crit Care Med 2004;32(4):916–21.
16. Barwaise A, Thongprayoon C, Gajic O, et al. Delayed rapid response team activation is associated with increased hospital mortality, morbidity, and length of stay in a Tertiary Care Institution. J Crit Care Med 2016;44(1):54–63.

17. Levy MM, Rhodes A, Phillips GS, et al. Surviving sepsis campaign: association between performeannce metrics and outcomes in a 7.5 year study. Crit Care Med 2015;43:3–12.

18. Thompson M, Reeves M, Bogan B, et al. Protocol- based resuscitation bundle to improve outcomes in septic shock patients: evaluation of the Michigan Health and Hospital Association keystone sepsis collaborative. Crit Care Med 2016; 44:2123–30.

19. ProCESS Investigators, Yealy DM, Kellum JA, Huang DT, et al. A randomized trial of protocol-based care for early septic shock. N Engl J Med 2014;370(18): 1683–93.

20. Guirgis FW, Jones L, Esma R, et al. Managing sepsis: electronic recognition, rapid response teams, and standardized care save lives. J Crit Care 2017;40: 296–302.

21. Seymour CW, Liu VX, Iwashyna TJ, et al. Assessment of clinical criteria for sepsis: for the Third International Consensus definitions for sepsis and septic shock (sepsis-3). JAMA 2016;315(8):762–74.

22. McBride J, Knight D, Piper J, et al. Long-term effect of introducing an early warning score on respiratory rate charting on general wards. Resuscitation 2005; 65(1):41–4.

Intensivist Presence at Code Events Is Associated with High Survival and Increased Documentation Rates

Mark Romig, MD[a],[*],[1], Jordan Duval-Arnould, MPH, DrPH[b],[1], Bradford D. Winters, PhD, MD[a], Heather Newton, BS, RN[c], Adam Sapirstein, MD[a]

KEYWORDS

- Cardiopulmonary resuscitation • Hospital rapid response team • Documentation
- Electronic health record

KEY POINTS

- Team leadership has been shown to be a significant factor in outcomes from cardiopulmonary arrest, and intensivist physicians are skilled in managing these crisis situations.
- Data assimilation from both integrated devices and provider documentation is necessary to support quality improvement efforts for cardiopulmonary arrest events.
- Attending intensivists can provide billable documentation which improves the ability to generate revenue to offset the cost of providing care at cardiopulmonary arrest events.

INTRODUCTION

In the United States, approximately 55% of all adult patients achieve return of spontaneous circulation (ROSC) following an in-hospital cardiac arrest and less than 25% survive to hospital discharge.[1–3] To improve outcomes, hospitals have employed emergency response teams, often referred as code teams, rapid response teams (RRTs), or medical emergency teams. Although RRTs have generally shown benefit through reductions in cardiopulmonary arrest (CPA) and in-hospital mortality, the factors associated with optimal rapid response system function are still being elucidated.[4] Some have hypothesized that team leadership may affect RRT effectiveness

[a] Johns Hopkins University, School of Medicine, Johns Hopkins Medicine, Armstrong Institute for Quality and Patient Safety, 1800 Orleans Street, Baltimore, MD 21287, USA; [b] Johns Hopkins University, School of Medicine, Johns Hopkins Medicine Simulation Center, 1800 Orleans Street, Baltimore, MD 21287, USA; [c] Resuscitation Events, Johns Hopkins Hospital, 1800 Orleans Street, Baltimore, MD 21287, USA
[1] These authors contributed equally to the work represented in this article.
* Corresponding author. 1800 Orleans Street, Meyer 297A, Baltimore, MD 21287.
E-mail address: mromig1@jhmi.edu

Crit Care Clin 34 (2018) 259–266
https://doi.org/10.1016/j.ccc.2017.12.009   criticalcare.theclinics.com

and patient outcome, but research on RRT leadership has generated conflicting results.[5,6]

To better support the highest function of the Johns Hopkins Hospital (JHH) adult code teams and RRTs, the authors created a team leadership role for a faculty intensivist. The International Liaison Committee on Resuscitation, the European Resuscitation Council, and the American Heart Association all recognize teamwork, communication, and leadership as significant factors in the performance of resuscitation teams.[7–9] The intention for this role was to integrate these elements and improve processes of care delivery, documentation, and decision-making. This article examines outcomes associated with the introduction of this role.

PROCESS

The JHH employs separate code teams and RRTs for adult medicine, surgery, and neurosciences. The composition of the RRT for each department is similar and employs an intensive care unit (ICU) charge nurse, a resident or fellow, and a nursing shift coordinator who are specific to the department. In addition, a pharmacist and respiratory therapist are notified of all RRT activations, but their presence is not mandatory and is driven by unit and ward demand.

Each department also maintains their own code team, which includes a member of the RRT and several other staff members. The medical intensive care senior resident is a member of all 3 code teams and responds to all events, regardless of department. In addition, a pharmacist and respiratory therapist are required to attend all code calls. A security officer responds to all code events to manage safety and coordinate expedited hospital transport if necessary.

In October of 2013, the central intensivist physician (CIP) was added as the team leader to all adult code team and RRT events. Before this time, the role of the CIP was largely operational because they performed ICU bed allocation and triage for patients requesting specialty surgical ICU and enhanced postoperative care.[10] Over time, the need to provide 24-hour support for allocation and triage of ICU services was identified. In addition, many requests for ICU care were generated following code team and RRT events. Therefore, the CIP role expanded in October 2013 to include (1) overnight coverage, (2) team leadership for all adult rapid response and code teams, and (3) consultation in 2 general surgical ICUs. Most important, the CIP serves as the airway management expert and critical care proceduralist at critical events.[11]

Before inclusion of the CIP on the code team, leadership varied based on the primary service caring for the patient (eg, medical vs surgical). None of the teams had dedicated attending level coverage and documentation of events varied based on the responding service.

Before July of 2017, there was no structured data collection tool in the electronic health record (EHR) for code-type events, therefore specific, identifiable documentation for code events was variable. Often, documentation consisted only of the resuscitation flow sheets and comments made by providers in progress notes. In July of 2017, the hospital deployed a combined code team and RRT note template within the Epic EHR (Epic Systems Corporation, Verona, WI, USA) and created a Code note type. The goals of these changes were to allow easy identification of specific event documentation and to standardize the entry of event data by the CIP. The JHH cardiopulmonary resuscitation (CPR) Committee's resuscitation science research group collects data and reviews performance of all code team and RRT events in the hospital. This information is used as part of a continuous learning model for resuscitation and to ensure that all phases of care meet current national standards. Analyses performed by the research group have been used to make inferences about the effectiveness of the CIP's leadership on the code teams and RTTs.

RESULTS

Approximately 40% of CPAs at JHH take place outside of a critical care location (**Fig. 1**) (median interquartile range [IQR]: ICU, 13 [10–19]; non-ICU, 9 [7–10]; $P<.001$). The leadership and technical roles for the CIP are likely to have the greatest value in this large number of CPAs.

The authors compared the survival to ROSC following CPA of greater than 20 minutes between events taking place in the ICU to those that took place outside of an ICU. **Fig. 2** is a control chart that shows that, after implementation of the CIP program, acute survival of the patients suffering CPA outside the ICU is equivalent to the survival of those in the ICU (ICU, 73.2% [64.3%–84.4%]; non-ICU, 73.0% [70.0%–90%]; $P = .51$).

The authors hypothesized that including code documentation as part of the responsibilities of the CIP would improve the quality of event documentation and that it would also be an indicator of the participation of the CIP in team management. We analyzed the documentation of non-ICU events by year and detected a significant improvement after creation of the EHR template. **Fig. 3** shows that, between the first and second program year, documentation significantly increased and variability decreased (2014, 88.3% [74.1]; 2015, 100% [95.1]; $P<.04$). This trend was maintained going forward. We bisected the program into the initial phase (January 2014–February 2015) and the subsequent phase (March 2015–June 2016) and found that the absolute number of events documented each month increased from 7 (IQR [3–9]) to 9 (IQR[8–10]) (**Fig. 4**).

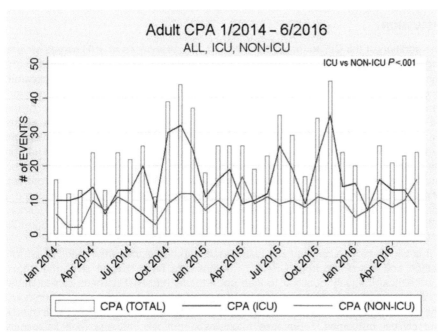

Fig. 1. Hospital location CPA events. The monthly total number of CPAs is shown by bars. Lines indicate events that occurred in an ICU (*red*) and outside the ICU (*green*).

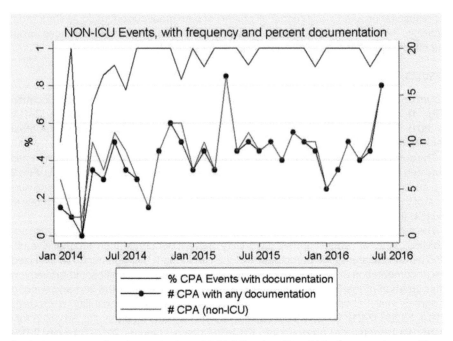

Fig. 2. Percentage of patients who have ROSC following CPA of 20 minutes or longer. There is no statistical difference in the acute survival following CPA of patients in an ICU (*blue line*) versus those not in the ICU (*red line*). ICU: 73.2% (64.3%–84.4%) versus non-ICU: 73.0% (70.0%–90%); $P = .51$.

DISCUSSION

The addition of the CIP to the code team and RRT responses at JHH serves several important functions. First, it provides attending physician supervision of airway management. Second, the CIP serves as a faculty consultant leader to the housestaff. Finally, the CIP documents the clinical events by completing both a formatted intervention template and a descriptive narrative summary. Before the addition of the CIP as the code team leader, attending-level physician involvement at code events was variable. Attending involvement was particularly scarce during the overnight and weekend periods when staffing is diminished. A CPA can occur anywhere in the hospital. When a CPA occurs in a critical care setting, it is rapidly recognized and the critical care team is equipped to begin resuscitation immediately. In contrast, when CPAs occur on the general wards at JHH, recognition may be delayed and a code team must be assembled by sending out emergency notifications. The authors believed that the greatest value of CIP leadership would be found in these non-ICU CPA events.

It is widely recognized that the team leadership has significant impact on performance and outcomes from CPA.[7–9,12] Intensivists have special skills that make them almost uniquely qualified to lead code teams and RRTs. These clinical situations may require directive, empowering, or both types of leadership techniques. The quality and type of leadership during resuscitations directly affects performance and clinical outcomes.[13] Because intensivists routinely manage multidisciplinary teams in crisis situations, they are trained and experienced in these leadership activities. In contrast, other faculty and house officers have highly variable leadership

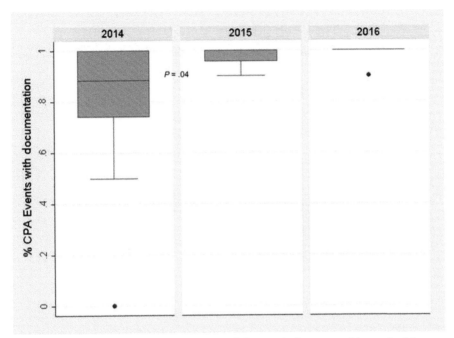

Fig. 3. Probability that a CPA event outside of the ICU is documented by a physician as a function of year. Physician documentation of CPA events was compared for each of the first 3 years of the program. Box plots show the percentage completion of CPA documentation by month. Boxes represent the middle interquartile ranges with divider bar at the mean. The outer quartiles are represented by the whiskers.

training and skills, even after they have completed resuscitation training.[14] Before the involvement of the CIP in the code team, leadership completely depended on the medical housestaff. Studies in both the Great Britain and Canada reveal that the housestaff often feel unprepared to lead CPA resuscitations.[12,15–20] The addition of the CIP allows senior housestaff at JHH to function to the level of their abilities and confidence, while providing them with an experienced consultant to ensure proper process and decision-making. Situation monitoring, mutual support, communication, and the ability to adapt are central team skills and the CIP role ensures these components, which, the authors believe, ultimately enhances the role of the senior residents.

Documentation of events that take place during a resuscitation is a key component of the learning health care system. Many of the required documentation elements may be captured in nursing flow sheets or through device integration. For example, the timing and quality of chest compressions is now electronically archived by the Johns Hopkins resuscitation science research group. However, not all required data is routinely recorded by these systems and these systems do not record clinical judgements or plans. Before the implementation of the CIP program, notes describing clinical events and clinicians' thinking were usually absent or of poor quality following code team and RRT events. There was, however, a meaningful increase in the physician documentation as the CIP program progressed. Although the hospital, through its CPR committee, had established required documentation metrics before the CIP, the authors believe that there was little knowledge among the housestaff (and others) about the need to meet

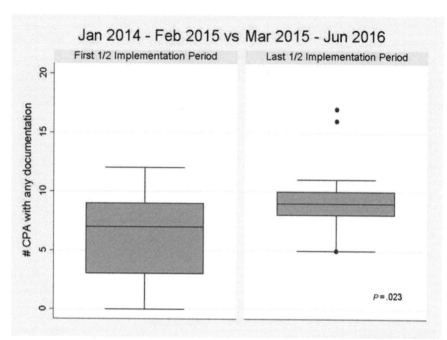

Fig. 4. Comparison of the number of non-ICU CPA events documented monthly in the first half and second half of the CIP program. The period during which the CIP program attended all code team and RRT events was divided into equal time periods with boxplots showing the number of monthly totals of CPA events with documentation. Boxes represent the middle interquartile ranges with divider bar at the mean. The outer quartiles are represented by the whiskers.

these requirements. This JHH case was likely similar to that found in Britain, where about 80% of house officers were unaware of nationally required resuscitation data entry.[14] Furthermore, many of the clinical insights at code team and RRT events are evanescent. Senior members of the resuscitation team often do not follow the patient longitudinally so that, failing documentation, their analysis may not contribute to ongoing patient care.

The addition of the CIP to the code team and the RRT also allows major operational efficiencies. Because the CIP performs ICU bed allocation and triage for all of the surgical services, he or she is able to rapidly transfer patients on the ward to ICU levels of care when needed. In addition, the CIP is able to assist in the initiation of critical care for all adult patients, irrespective of their service. Although there are no data about the clinical benefits of these interventions, the authors believe that the CIP has significantly decreased the time from recognition to increased level of care for critically ill patients following both code team and RRT events. In addition, when no attending physician was supervising resuscitations, the hospital did not submit bills for CPR. Because of the need to constitute, equip, and perform quality assurance for several teams, the cost of resuscitation services is high. The authors estimate that $57,000 per year can be generated by the CIP in JHH through proper professional billing for CPR alone (average reimbursement of $176, with 27 events per month). This figure is likely to be much higher when additional billing for other procedures and critical care services is included. This revenue is important because it provides financing for attending-level staffing and supports the team efforts of the

JHH. The ability to bill for these events improves documentation quality and compliance because clinical records are administratively reviewed to assure that they support appropriate billing.

Although it is plausible that attending intensivist presence at a code event improves outcomes after cardiac arrest, there are inadequate data to conclusively prove this hypothesis. Indeed, the CIP is only 1 component in the quality improvement and data collection arms of the RRT program that have taken place at JHH over the last few years. At the same time, improvement in documentation would not be possible without the presence of an attending physician.

There are a variety of staffing models for RRTs and code teams. Nurses, resident physicians, nurse practitioners, and physician assistants may function as team leaders, as opposed to attending physicians. There has been no outcome benefit demonstrated among the various leadership models. However, unlike other models, the CIP is able to provide hospital administrative leadership, critical care procedural expertise, and revenue capture through billing. Although other leadership models may have some combination of these advantages, only an attending physician–driven model is able to meet all these needs.

SUMMARY

Since expanding the role of the central intensivist to include overnight coverage 6 days per week, there has been improvement in RRT and code documentation, thus providing data for quality improvement and perhaps improving continuity of care for patients. During this same period, there has been improvement in ROSC after cardiac arrest, suggesting CIP impact.

Health care systems designing the composition of their RRTs and code teams must make a value judgment about the cost of staffing versus the potential benefit they provide. To date, the only other articles to consider the role of intensivists as team members were not designed explicitly examine the effect of intensivist presence and were limited to only considering patient outcome.[5,6] This article demonstrates that an intensivist has the potential to improve patient care while offsetting costs through improved billing capture.

REFERENCES

1. Peberdy MA, Kaye W, Ornato JP, et al. Cardiopulmonary resuscitation of adults in the hospital: a report of 14720 cardiac arrests from the National Registry of Cardiopulmonary Resuscitation. Resuscitation 2003;58:297–308.
2. Chan P. Public health burden of in-hospital cardiac arrest. Washington, DC: Institute of Medicine; 2015.
3. Girotra S, Nallamothu BK, Spertus JA, et al. Trends in survival after in-hospital cardiac arrest. N Engl J Med 2012;367:1912–20.
4. Winters BD, Weaver SJ, Pfoh ER, et al. Rapid-response systems as a patient safety strategy: a systematic review. Ann Intern Med 2013;158:417–25.
5. Bannard-Smith J, Lighthall GK, Subbe CP, et al. Clinical outcomes of patients seen by rapid response teams: a template for benchmarking international teams. Resuscitation 2016;107:7–12.
6. Scherr K, Wilson DM, Wagner J, et al. Evaluating a new rapid response team: NP-led versus intensivist-led comparisons. AACN Adv Crit Care 2012;23:32–42.
7. Bhanji F, Mancini ME, Sinz E, et al. Part 16: education, implementation, and teams: 2010 American Heart Association guidelines for cardiopulmonary resuscitation and emergency cardiovascular care. Circulation 2010;122:S920–33.

8. Mancini ME, Soar J, Bhanji F, et al. Part 12: education, implementation, and teams: 2010 International consensus on cardiopulmonary resuscitation and emergency cardiovascular care science with treatment recommendations. Circulation 2010;122:S539–81.

9. Nolan JP, Soar J, Zideman DA, et al. European resuscitation council guidelines for resuscitation 2010 section 1. Executive summary. Resuscitation 2010;81: 1219–76.

10. Romig M, Latif A, Pronovost P, et al. Centralized triage for multiple intensive care units: the central intensivist physician. Am J Med Qual 2010;25:343–5.

11. Mark LJ, Herzer KR, Cover R, et al. Difficult airway response team: a novel quality improvement program for managing hospital-wide airway emergencies. Anesth Analg 2015;121:127–39.

12. Yeung JH, Ong GJ, Davies RP, et al. Factors affecting team leadership skills and their relationship with quality of cardiopulmonary resuscitation. Crit Care Med 2012;40:2617–21.

13. Ford K, Menchine M, Burner E, et al. Leadership and teamwork in trauma and resuscitation. West J Emerg Med 2016;17:549–56.

14. Robinson PS, Shall E, Rakhit R. Cardiac arrest leadership: in need of resuscitation? Postgrad Med J 2016;92:715–20.

15. Hayes CW, Rhee A, Detsky ME, et al. Residents feel unprepared and unsupervised as leaders of cardiac arrest teams in teaching hospitals: a survey of internal medicine residents. Crit Care Med 2007;35:1668–72.

16. Merchant RM, Berg RA, Yang L, et al. Hospital variation in survival after in-hospital cardiac arrest. J Am Heart Assoc 2014;3:e000400.

17. Henriksen K, Battles J, Keyes M, et al. Advances in patient safety: new directions and alternative approaches. Rockville (MD): Agency for Healthcare Research and Quality; 2008.

18. Cannon-Bowers J, Salas E. Teamwork competencies: the interaction of team member knowledge, skills, and attitudes. In: O'Neil HF Jr, editor. Workforce readiness: competencies and assessment. Mahwah: Lawrence Erlbaum Associates; 1997. p. 151–74.

19. Smith-Jentsch K, Baker D, Salas E, et al. Uncovering differences in team competency requirements: the case of air traffic control teams. In: Salas E, Bowers C, Edens E, editors. Improving teamwork in organizations: applications of resource management training. Mahwah: Lawrence Erlbaum Associates; 2001. p. 31–54.

20. Seamster T, Kaempf G. Identifying resource management skills for airline pilots. In: Salas E, Bowers C, Edens E, editors. Improving teamwork in organizations: applications of resource management training. Mahwah: Lawrence Erlbaum Associates; 2001. p. 9–30.

Section II: Fluid Resuscitation

Edited By: Andrew D. Shaw and
Sean M. Bagshaw

Preface

Fluid Therapy in the Critically Ill

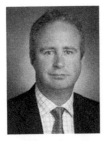 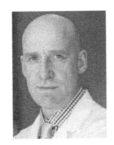

Andrew D. Shaw, MB, FRCA,   Sean M. Bagshaw, MD, MSc, FRCPC
FFICM, FCCM, MMHC

Editors

The debate about how much fluid to give to intensive care unit (ICU) patients, and what type, rages on and has done so for over a century. This debate is typical of any medical controversy—fueled by emotional attachment and cognitive bias to a lifetime's practice and not encumbered by any firm evidence-based guidelines. Crystalloid or colloid? Synthetic or blood product–derived colloid? Blood or no blood and if so at what threshold to transfuse? High or low chloride? Is 0.9% saline bad for you? Is it ever good? How much before the hazard becomes clinically apparent? How can colloid be good for you in the operating room/theater environment but bad for you in the ICU?

AMOUNT OF FLUID

It is probably generally agreed that too much fluid is bad for critically ill patients. The problem is that in practice it is very difficult not to give these patients intravenous (IV) fluids, especially when the blood pressure is low or the urine output is deemed inadequate. We do know from several large observational studies that critically ill patients who accumulate a positive fluid balance over the course of their ICU stay tend to experience worse long-term outcomes than patients who are kept in even fluid balance, or in whom fluids are more conservatively managed. Critics of these studies argue they merely represent patients of different complexity and severity, while supporters of fluid restriction argue that oxygen flux in tissues and organs is better maintained by minimizing extracellular fluid accumulation.

TYPE OF FLUID: COLLOID

The intraoperative goal-directed fluid literature clearly supports protocolized administration of colloidal solutions for volume optimization, particularly in the context of colorectal surgery, and as part of an enhanced recovery program. Whether this concept can be extended to other types of major surgery, and how sick patients can be included in these programs, is less clear. Furthermore, failure to accept that a given patient is not progressing along the "fast track" and changing strategy has been associated with increased morbidity. It is clear that one size does not fit all in this context. Synthetic or natural colloids have both been used for intraoperative goal directed therapy, and a clear advantage of one over the other has not been demonstrated. Last, whether goal directed therapy can be achieved using crystalloid solutions has still not been convincingly demonstrated or refuted.

TYPE OF FLUID: CRYSTALLOID

Recently, much attention has been directed to the issue of physiologically balanced versus unbalanced crystalloid solutions in the context of IV fluid therapy. There are several large studies in both surgical and medical populations, suggesting that there may be a morbidity and mortality hazard associated with the use of 0.9% saline, although this has not yet been convincingly proven in large randomized trials. Whether it actually needs to be proven is a matter of debate, and some would argue that when there is no clear benefit, no significant price differential, and a probable harm, then that would signal that the practice should change anyway.

SUMMARY

As we move to an era where payers, patients, and health care professionals are focusing on health rather than care, it will be increasingly important to identify those therapies and treatments that are the most cost-effective and the least harmful. IV fluid is the commonest inpatient intervention, and as such, the population at risk is enormous. Even small differences between types of fluid are thus important to identify, and if we fail to do so, then we will effectively be failing in our primary responsibility to our patients: primum non nocere.

Andrew D. Shaw, MB, FRCA, FFICM, FCCM, MMHC
Department of Anesthesiology and Pain Medicine
University of Alberta
2-150 Clinical Sciences Building
Edmonton, Alberta T6G 2G3, Canada

Sean M. Bagshaw, MD, MSc, FRCPC
Department of Critical Care Medicine
University of Alberta
2-124 Clinical Sciences Building
Edmonton, Alberta T6G 2B7, Canada

E-mail addresses:
ashaw2@ualberta.ca (A.D. Shaw)
bagshaw@ualberta.ca (S.M. Bagshaw)

Applied Physiology of Fluid Resuscitation in Critical Illness

Sabrina Arshed, MD, Michael R. Pinsky, MD, CM, Dr hc*

KEYWORDS

- Effective circulating blood volume • Mean systemic pressure • Venous return
- Stressed volume • Unstressed volume

KEY POINTS

- Venous return defines cardiac output.
- Fluid resuscitation aims to increase mean systemic pressure.
- Both fluids and vasopressors can increase mean systemic pressure and cardiac output.
- Crystalloids distribute across the body, whereas colloids tend to remain intravascular longer.

INTRODUCTION

Cardiovascular instability presenting as hypotension is often associated with decreased effective circulating blood volume and an associated increase in sympathetic tone. In the past, fluid management was the initial treatment of choice for all causes of hypotension. Although fluid management remains controversial, it is generally now agreed that fluids are not a 1-size fits all therapy; rather, it is a tailored management because the goals of care differ based on the cause of cardiovascular collapse. Indeed, many different processes can result in cardiovascular instability, not all of which benefit from fluid resuscitation. Only those patients in whom increasing the mean systemic pressure (Pms) will increase cardiac output are treated with fluid infusions. In the setting of trauma, the mechanism of cardiovascular instability is often hypovolemia secondary to hemorrhage; whereas in sepsis, the initial mechanism is increased unstressed blood volume due to a generalized inflammatory response-induced vasoplegia. However, with massive pulmonary embolism, cardiovascular

Disclosure Statement: The authors have no commercial interests related to the content of this article.
Department of Critical Care Medicine, University of Pittsburgh, 1215.4 Kaufmann Medical Building, 3471 Fifth Avenue, Pittsburgh, PA 15213, USA
* Corresponding author.
E-mail address: pinsky@pitt.edu

Crit Care Clin 34 (2018) 267–277
https://doi.org/10.1016/j.ccc.2017.12.010
0749-0704/18/© 2017 Elsevier Inc. All rights reserved.

instability is caused by right ventricular (RV) failure due to pulmonary vascular obstruction; in myocardial infarction, it is caused by decreased systolic pump function. Neither of these 2 common causes of circulatory shock is effectively treated by fluid infusion. To illustrate this, this article reviews the determinants of cardiac output, then the various shock causes, and then the fluids used to treat them.

CARDIOVASCULAR PHYSIOLOGY 101
Why Give Fluids?

In cardiovascular resuscitation, the only reason to give fluids is to increase the Pms in the hope that it will increase the pressure gradient for venous return, thereby increasing cardiac output. Because the back pressure to venous return is right atrial pressure (Pra) and because the heart can only pump the blood it receives, it should be clear that the primary job of the heart with regard to cardiac output is to keep the Pra as low as possible so as to optimize this pressure gradient. Indeed, cardiogenic and obstructive shock can rapidly lead to cardiovascular collapse because the associated sudden increases in the Pra impair venous return and thus impede left ventricular (LV) filling, such that cardiac output and arterial pressure decrease. These points are illustrated on the combined LV function and venous return curves if one plots cardiac output verses the Pra (**Fig. 1**).

Effective Circulating Blood Volume

The Pms reflects the impact of blood volume distribution on the subsequent stressed volume of the circulation. However, most of the circulating blood volume, although it fills the intravascular spaces, does not directly contribute to the Pms. If one were to take a circularity system, otherwise intact but devoid of volume, and start infusing whole blood into the vascular space, a curious thing would happen: nothing. Venous pressures would remain at 0 and no flow would come back to the heart to allow pumping, even though quite a lot of blood might have been initially infused. Eventually, after enough blood was infused into the circulation, equal to approximately 60% to 70% of the total circulatory blood volume, another curious thing would occur: on infusion of

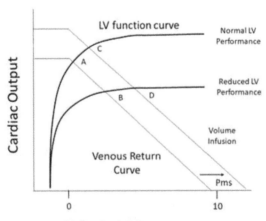

Fig. 1. Relationship between LV contractility (lines A–C and B–D) and intravascular volume changes on venous return (lines A–B and C–D). Fluid resuscitation increases Pms which on this graph is the Pra at the zero cardiac output value.

just a little bit more fluid, the Pms would rapidly increase. This would be because the blood would have finally distended the vessels enough to cause them to require their walls to stretch to further increase their intravascular volume, instead of just altering their shape. This tipping point represents the blood volume exceeding the unstressed volume and causing the Pms to increase, thus creating an upstream pressure that may allow venous return to start. Vascular compliance is usually measured as the change in the Pms to the change in blood volume above the unstressed volume. Importantly, only small amounts of fluid are needed to vary the Pms above this unstressed volume. This venous unstressed volume's transmural pressure is, by definition, zero, and it does not directly contribute to the upstream pressure driving venous return.[1,2] Most of the circulating blood volume resides in the venous portion of the systemic circulation. Venous vascular beds contain approximately 70% of the body's blood volume, consisting of unstressed (70%) and stressed (30%) volume (see previous description).[1] Stressed venous volume represents blood volume in excess of the unstressed volume and its volume to venomotor tone defines the Pms, the upstream pressure for venous return.[2] Unstressed volume can be rapidly varied by the host by simply altering blood flow distribution away from high capacitance (high unstressed volume) vessels, such as the splanchnic circulation, to cause the Pms to increase, or altering it toward these vessels to allow the Pms to decrease. Under normal conditions, the body's ability to rapidly vary unstressed volume is the primary means by which it alters venous return (cardiac output) in response to varying metabolic demands. Importantly, the blood volume below the unstressed volume is only a theoretic volume because all blood contributes to circulation once the Pms exceeds 0.

Similarly, acute adrenergic excess, such as during a massive intracranial hemorrhage, can cause hydrostatic pulmonary edema even though total blood volume is unchanged because unstressed blood volume decreases; whereas in sepsis unstressed volume increases as more parallel vascular circuits are dilated and their vascular beds perfused. Although alterations in sympathetic tone and vasoplegia can also markedly alter the resistance to venous return, defined as the ratio of the difference between the Pms and the Pra to cardiac output, fluid resuscitation by itself rarely causes large changes in the resistance to venous return.

All examples of circulatory shock (see later discussion) illustrate how changes in sympathetic tone, vascular responsiveness, or its lack (vasoplegia), as well as changes in the Pra, influence the impact of fluid infusion on cardiac output and arterial pressure. Thus, shock states can decrease the Pms by increasing unstressed volume (eg, sepsis), decreasing total blood volume (eg, hemorrhage), or decreasing the pressure gradient for venous return (eg, pulmonary embolism or heart failure).

Acute Cardiogenic Shock

Acute cardiogenic shock is defined as acute heart failure with a systolic arterial pressure less than 90 mm Hg and hypoperfusion. The end-organ hypoperfusion is due to the combined effects of severe reduction in cardiac index, causing arterial hypotension and elevated cardiac filling pressures, and increasing venous pressure.[3] The lack of forward flow results in pulmonary edema. The major problem surrounding cardiogenic shock is that the failing heart needs fluid but an often preexisting diastolic dysfunction makes the heart incredibly sensitive to fluid.

The difficulty in the management of cardiogenic shock is maintaining mean arterial pressures adequate enough to support coronary perfusion while minimizing LV afterload. Clearly, treatments directed at reversing coronary artery insufficiency are central to the etiologic management of acute heart failure but are independent of these other therapeutic considerations. Given the severe reduction in cardiac index with elevated filling pressures, pulmonary edema is a common sequela of cardiogenic shock, often treated with furosemide, leading to hypovolemia in a previously euvolemic patient. More focused therapy would include measures aimed at minimizing LV afterload while preserving coronary blood flow. Currently, only 2 therapies accomplish these goals: intraaortic balloon counter-pulsation and continuous positive airway pressure ventilatory support. Within this context, fluid resuscitation is problematic and, if given, needs to be given cautiously because of the risk of LV overdistention.

Current pharmacologic therapies for cardiogenic shock are vasopressors and inotropes. Vasopressors should be avoided because they are associated with poor outcomes in cardiogenic shock.[4] Inotropic agents are often used in the setting of acute cardiogenic shock; however, they increase myocardial adenosine triphosphate consumption, resulting in transient hemodynamic improvement at the expense of increased oxygen demand of the failing heart.[5] Although fluid resuscitation remains controversial in the setting of acute cardiogenic pulmonary edema, it may be effective when administered in small judicious volumes with close invasive hemodynamic or echocardiographic monitoring to restore coronary perfusion pressure without overdistention.

Obstructive Shock

Obstructive shock is the end product of either impaired ventricular filling or ejection, independent of myocardial contractility. It results in a reduction in cardiac output with normal or increased (if chronic) intravascular volume and myocardial function.[6] Examples of obstructive shock include pericardial tamponade, which directly impairs diastolic filling of the right ventricle; tension pneumothorax; and lung hyperinflation, which obstructs venous return, indirectly impairing RV filling.[6] However, the most common cause of acute obstructive shock is a massive pulmonary embolism.

Massive pulmonary emboli carry a high level of morbidity and mortality. However, the severity of acute pulmonary embolism is often determined by its hemodynamic impact, specifically the development of acute pulmonary hypertension. Acute pulmonary hypertension leads to an increase in RV afterload and RV dilatation, leading to right heart failure through a variety of interrelated mechanisms.[7] Acute RV dilation immediately decreases LV diastolic compliance by the process of ventricular interdependence. In essence, there is only so much volume inside the pericardium and, if the right ventricle is dilated, the left ventricle has no room to passively fill in diastole.[8] Thus, LV stroke volume decreases and hypotension ensues, causing RV ischemia, which combines with dilation to cause acute cor pulmonale. Clearly, in this setting, rapid fluid resuscitation is contraindicated because it will only make RV dilation worse; however, no fluid in the setting of increased RV afterload is also inadequate. Thus, how much volume to give a patient in acute cor pulmonale is extremely difficult to define as an isolated therapy and needs to be done in concert with vasopressors and, potentially, inotropes.

The dilated right ventricle in the setting of a massive pulmonary embolism is extremely fluid insensitive in terms of changes in end-diastolic volume but very fluid-sensitive in terms of changes in filling pressure. Overresuscitation with intravenous fluids will lead to the rapid development of both cor pulmonale and venous hypertension. Earlier studies reported that an increase in cardiac output was inversely proportional to RV dilatation before fluid expansion in patients with pulmonary emboli.[9] This suggests rapid fluid resuscitation can be detrimental due to increasing RV stress and subsequent decrease in cardiac output and cardiovascular collapse. However, if fluids are necessary, they must be administered in small amounts under echocardiographic monitoring to identify early signs of paradoxic septal shift and/or tricuspid regurgitation.

Hemorrhagic Shock

Acute traumatic injury is the most common cause of hemorrhagic shock, due to both acute blood loss and trauma-induced coagulopathy. It is imperative to restore circulatory blood volume and repair large arterial lesions. Fluid resuscitation is the primary therapy in traumatic hemorrhagic shock. However, resuscitation with large volumes of crystalloids can lead to interstitial edema and abdominal compartment syndrome.[10] Usually, if the blood loss is rapid, whole blood resuscitation improves outcomes. However, if bleeding is subacute, even if massive, fluid resuscitation is often effective at restoring cardiovascular sufficiency despite a lowering of hematocrit.

The cause of continued hypovolemia in trauma patients is complex. Clearly, failure of tie off arterial bleeding sites causes continual volume loss but so does trauma-induced coagulopathy. Trauma-induced coagulopathy is common in traumatic hemorrhagic shock, with 10% to 34% of patients developing coagulopathy.[11,12] The causes of the coagulopathy are delusional, consumption, and endothelial dysfunction. Plasma and red blood cells should be transfused as soon as possible in traumatic hemorrhagic shock patients to maintain sufficient oxygen delivery and restore effective coagulation.

The optimal plasma to red blood cell ratio remains highly controversial; however, due to the high mortality of trauma-induced coagulopathy, several trauma centers have advocated using a plasma to red blood cell ratio of 1 to 1.[13] Furthermore, a few large trauma centers across the United States have started using uncrossed whole blood, the resuscitative fluid of choice in traumatic hemorrhagic shock, in the emergency department trauma bay.

Distributive Shock

Distributive shock results from vasoplegia and impaired distribution of blood flow.[14] Distributive shock is different from other forms of shock, in that the fluid resuscitation strategy is not simple. Sustained trauma, sepsis, and the postoperative state are all examples of distributive shock due to their vasoplegic state. However, the most common clinical cause of distributive shock is septic shock.

In septic shock, the initial effect is a generalized inflammatory shock, leading to vasoplegia, which is a condition of low systemic vascular resistance due to impaired vascular smooth muscle response to adrenergic stimulation. In fact, circulating levels of norepinephrine are increased in most patients who are in septic shock. The pathophysiology of septic shock is complex, complicated by venodilation, capillary leak, and vasoplegia. Septic vasoplegia leads to an increase in unstressed volume decreasing the Pms because many previously nonperfused vascular beds receive blood flow, whereas the resistance to venous return also increases as hepatic vascular tone is transiently increased. Thus, the Pms often decreases early in sepsis due to increased unstressed volume. Thus, these patients need fluid resuscitation even if they have not lost any volume through edema formation because their unstressed volume increases because of the increased total number of vascular beds, independent of their metabolic needs. Furthermore, with the generalized intravascular inflammatory response, there can be both decrease in capillary perfused density[15] and decreased barrier function, allowing greater extravasation of fluid from the capillary into the interstitium. This capillary leakage causes both hypovolemia and decreased capillary hydrostatic pressure.[15] For this reason, aggressive fluid resuscitation is recommended in early sepsis to restore microcirculation and normalize the capillary hydrostatic pressure to promote tissue perfusion.[16] However, when the capillary hydrostatic pressure has been normalized, further fluid resuscitation may lead to hypervolemia, peripheral edema, and increased mortality.[17] Finally, the loss of vascular tone, or vasoplegia, is thought to be due to a combination of endothelial injury by oxidative stress, vasopressin deficiency, release of inflammatory mediators, and inactivation of catecholamines.[18,19] In the setting of vasoplegia, normal autoregulation makes blood flow ineffective, requiring progressively increasing cardiac output to maintain adequate oxygen delivery to tissues. All of the previously mentioned factors combine in septic shock, leading to a refractory shock with poor outcomes.

FLUIDS

In the past, clinicians based their resuscitation fluid preference on the idea of fluid compartments, specifically the intracellular and extracellular compartments, with the extracellular compartment comprising intravascular and interstitial spaces.[20] The semipermeable membranes of the extracellular compartment in conjunction with oncotic and hydrostatic pressures were the factors of transvascular fluid exchange.

However, recent evidence favors a negatively charged meshwork of biopolymers, which coat the endothelium, known as the endothelial glycocalyx[21] (**Fig. 2**). The endothelial glycocalyx plays an important role in the movement of fluids and solutes across membranes. The subglycocalyx space produces a colloid oncotic pressure, which determines transcapillary flow.[22] Nonfenestrated capillaries have been identified within the interstitial space, indicating that fluid from the interstitium is returned to the

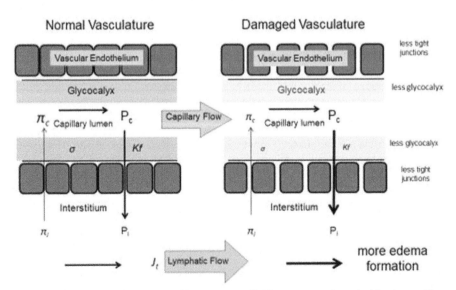

Starling Forces and Fluid Flux Across the Capillary Endothelial Barrier

Fig. 2. The forces acting in the capillary to cause fluid movement from inside the capillary lumen into the interstitium or vice versa. π, oncotic pressure; σ, reflection coefficient; Kf, filtration coefficient; J_t, lymphatic flow. (*Adapted from* Lira A, Pinsky MR. Choices in fluid type and volume during resuscitation: impact on patient outcomes. Ann Intensive Care 2014;4:38; with permission.)

circulation primarily as lymph, via several large pores.[22] The extent that vascular endo-thelial intercellular tight junctions are disrupted or that glycocalyx loss predominates in creating increased capillary permeability is still in debate.

The endothelial glycocalyx is fairly stable under physiologic conditions; however, degradation can be linked to inflammation, capillary leakage, and disease states, such as ischemia-reperfusion injury, sepsis, and trauma.[23] Once damaged, the endo-thelial glycocalyx restoration can take several days. Based on these concepts, clini-cians often give fluids based on their presumed volume of distribution. Colloids are thought to remain intravascularly longer and crystalloids tend to distribute better in to-tal body water. If intravascular volume loss has taken more than a few hours, gener-alized volume loss occurs and crystalloids should be given to restore interstitial and cellular volumes. However, if volume loss is very rapid, as in massive hemorrhage or anaphylaxis, colloids will retain intravascular volume and thus sustain a higher Pms during acute resuscitation.

Intravascular fluids can divided into crystalloids and colloids based on their molec-ular composition (**Table 1**). Colloids have a high-molecular-weight molecule as part of their solution, which limits the rapid efflux of volume from the intervascular space into the interstitium. Colloids are merely crystalloid solutions with colloids added to them. Both the nature of the electrolytes used in each and the nature of the colloids affect their effectiveness and complication rates.

CRYSTALLOIDS

There are essentially 3 categories of crystalloid fluids: glucose in water with or without electrolytes, the variations of saline, and the balanced salt solutions. The use of salt-based fluid resuscitation dates back to the cholera pandemic of the 1830s, when Dr. Robert Lewins[24] successfully resuscitated 6 patients with a sodium chloride (NaCl)-based solution. Thus, began a 200-year streak of resuscitation with so-called normal saline. This is a misnomer because there is nothing normal about normal saline; 0.9% NaCl contains 154 mEq/L of sodium and 154 mEq/L of chloride, which is exceedingly supraphysiologic to extracellular fluid.[25] In addition, its low pH, and lack of potassium, bicarbonate, calcium, magnesium, and phosphorous may elicit metabolic acidosis and hyperchloremia, causing renal vasoconstriction and promoting acute kidney injury and secretion of inflammatory cytokines.[25–27] The only physiologic indication for using 0.9% NaCl solutions is to treat hypochloremic metabolic alkalosis, a side effect of excessive diuretic use.

Use of a more physiologic crystalloid solution for resuscitation is associated with increased survivorship and less kidney injury. Such balanced salt solutions include lactated Ringer or Plasma-Lyte. Several large observational studies have demon-strated superior outcomes with the use of balanced fluids.[28,29] Nonetheless, balanced salt solutions are relatively hypotonic (lactated Ringer sodium 131 mEq/L, Plasma-Lyte sodium 130 mEq/L).[26] Excessive administration of balanced solutions may result in metabolic alkalosis, hyperlactatemia, or hypotonicity.[20] However, given the concern regarding excess sodium and chloride, balanced salt solutions are the resuscitation crystalloids of choice.

In addition, there has been concern regarding the extravasation of crystalloids in to the interstitial space during aggressive resuscitation. In the setting of trauma, fluid resuscitation is directly replacing intravascular losses, thus the goal is to use fluids that will remain in the intravascular space. However, in the setting of vasoplegia, there has been endothelial glycocalyx damage and fluid absorption is essentially taking place in the subglycocalyx, located within the interstitial space.[22] Therefore, fluid

Table 1
Examples of commercially available crystalloid and colloid solutions

Solute	Plasma	Colloids				Crystalloids		
		4% Albumin	6% HES 130/0.4	Dextran	Gelatin	Normal Saline	Ringer Lactate	Plasma-Lyte
Sodium (Na^+)	135–145	148	154	154	154	154	130	140
Potassium (K^+)	4.0–5.0	0	0	0	0	0	4.5	5
Calcium (Ca^{+2})	2.2–2.6	0	0	0	0	0	2.7	0
Magnesium (Mg^{+2})	1.0–2.0	0	0	0	0	0	0	1.5
Chlorine (Cl)$^-$	95–110	128	154	154	120	154	109	98
Acetate	0	0	0	0	0	0	0	27
Lactate	0.8–1.8	0	0	0	0	0	28	0
Gluconate	0	0	0	0	0	0	0	23
Bicarb	23–26	0	0	0	0	0	0	0
Osmolarity	291	250	286–308	308	274	308	280	294
Colloid	35–45	20	60	100	40	0	0	0

Osmolarity (mOsm/L); Colloid (g/L); all other solutes (mmol/L).

extravasation into the interstitium is not only expected, it is hoped, to maintain cardiac output and maintain adequate oxygen delivery. Nonetheless, in a study comparing crystalloids to albumin,[30] the only group that had a survival advantage from albumin over crystalloids was the group of subjects in sepsis shock.

COLLOIDS

Colloids are a class of high-molecular-weight compounds that confer oncotic pressure, thus allowing them to remain longer in the intravascular space under normal physiologic conditions.[20] Albumin is the most commonly used colloid currently used in North America. In Europe, hydroxyethyl starch (HES) is more commonly used, especially during surgery, though use is decreasing. HES has been linked to acute kidney injury in septic patients and its use in those patients has been banned in Europe and not recommended in the surviving sepsis guidelines.[31] The final colloid is gelatin, made from horses' hoofs. Gelatins remain available outside of North America but are not available in North America because of their slight (1 per 1000) incidence of anaphylaxis.

Human albumin has been the most widely studied colloid as a resuscitation fluid in the critically ill. Under normal conditions it is synthesized by the liver and is responsible for 80% of intravascular colloid oncotic pressure.[32] In 2004, the Saline versus Albumin Fluid Evaluation (SAFE) trial compared 4% albumin with normal saline for fluid resuscitation in the intensive care unit. No difference was found between the 2 groups for the primary endpoint of 28-day all-cause mortality.[33] However, in patients with traumatic brain injuries, the relative risk of death was greater with albumin when compared with saline. This is thought to be due to a coagulation defect induced by albumin.[33,34] However, in the SAFE trial, subjects with sepsis and septic shock who received albumin had an adjusted relative risk of death at 28 days of 0.71; suggesting a beneficial effect.[33] In the ALBIOS study, albumin was compared with normal saline in the management of subjects in circulatory shock.[30] The only group in which outcomes were better with albumin was the group in which the subjects were in septic shock, suggesting that specific patients' albumin still has a place in resuscitation.

Starches are a group of semisynthetic colloids from sorghum corn or potatoes, which are classified based on their weight and the number of hydroxyethyl groups per glucose monomer.[20] First-generation and second-generation starches used higher molecular weight with larger numbers of hydroxyethyl groups, which, in turn, lengthened the duration of intravascular volume expansion.[35] Unfortunately, this was at the expense of alterations to coagulation patterns and accumulation in the kidneys, leading to acute kidney injury.[20]

Third-generation starches, or the modern HES, have lower molecular weights and reduced numbers of hydroxyethyl groups, which is thought to lead to less toxicity.[35] They are less expensive and easier to produce than albumin. In 2012, the Crystalloid versus Hydroxyethyl Starch Trial (CHEST) compared 6% HES to 0.9% saline in critically ill adults requiring fluid resuscitation.[31] There was no difference in the primary outcome of 90-day all-cause mortality between the 2 groups. However, subjects randomized to the HES group experienced a doubling in the incidence of treatment-related adverse events, specifically skin rash, pruritus, and acute kidney injury.[31] Despite numerous subsequent trials, there is no convincing evidence to suggest the superiority of HES over other fluid resuscitation strategies in critically ill patients.

SUMMARY

In conclusion, fluid resuscitation of the critically ill patient is quite complex. Previous clinical habits based on tradition used normal saline in large boluses for all causes of hypotension. Although fluid management remains controversial, balanced salt solutions remain the resuscitative fluid of choice in most conditions. Furthermore, just as the cause of cardiovascular collapse differs patient to patient, so do their needs for fluid and the amount of fluid, if given. Treatment and resuscitative strategies are still a bedside art, not just a fixed resuscitation protocol.

REFERENCES

1. Gelman S. Venous function and central venous pressure. Anesthesiology 2008; 108:735–48.
2. Broccard AF. Cardiopulmonary interactions and volume status assessment. J Clin Monit Comput 2012;26:383–91.
3. Reynolds HR, Hochman JS. Cardiogenic shock: current concepts and improving outcomes. Circulation 2008;117(5):686–97.
4. Valente S, Lazzeri C, Vecchio S, et al. Predictors of in-hospital mortality after percutaneous coronary intervention for cardiogenic shock. Int J Cardiol 2007; 114:176–82.
5. Mebazaa A, Nieminen MS, Packer M, et al. Levosimendan vs dobutamine for patients with acute decompensated heart failure: the SURVIVE randomized trial. JAMA 2007;297:1883–91.
6. Kumar A, Parillo JE. Shock: classification, pathophysiology, and approach to management. In: Parillo JE, Dellinger RP, editors. Critical care medicine: principles of diagnosis and management in the adult. 3rd edition. Philadelphia: Mosby Elsevier; 2008. p. 379–422.
7. Belohlavek J, Dytrych V, Linhart A. Pulmonary embolism part I: epidemiology, risk factors and risk stratification, pathophysiology, clinical presentation, diagnosis and nonthrombotic pulmonary embolism. Exp Clin Cardiol 2013;18(2):129–38.
8. Grifoni S, Olivotto I, Cecchini P, et al. Short-term clinical outcome of patients with acute pulmonary embolism, normal blood pressure, and echocardiographic right ventricular dysfunction. Circulation 2000;101:2817–22.
9. Meyer G, Vieillard-Baron A, Planquette B. Recent advances in the management of pulmonary embolism: focus on the critically ill patients. Ann Intensive Care 2016;6:19.
10. Madigan MC, Kemp CD, Johnson JC, et al. Secondary abdominal compartment syndrome after severe extremity injury: are early, aggressive fluid resuscitation strategies to blame? J Trauma 2008;64:280–5.
11. Brohi K, Cohen MJ, Davenport RA. Acute coagulopathy of trauma: mechanism, identification and effect. Curr Opin Crit Care 2007;13:680–5.
12. Brohi K, Cohen MJ, Ganter MT, et al. Acute coagulopathy of trauma: hypoperfusion induces systemic anticoagulation and hyperfibrinolysis. J Trauma 2008;64: 1211–7.
13. Moore EE, Chin TL, Chapman MC, et al. Plasma first in the field for postinjury hemorrhagic shock. Shock 2014;41(1):35–8.
14. Levy MM, Fink MP, Marshall JC, et al. 2001 SCCM/ESICM/ACCP/ATS/SIS international sepsis definitions conference. Crit Care Med 2003;31(4):1250–6.
15. De Backer D, Ospina-Tascon G, Salgado D, et al. Monitoring the microcirculation in the critically ill patient: current methods and future approaches. Intensive Care Med 2010;36:1813–25.
16. Tatara T. Context-sensitive fluid therapy in critical illness. J Intensive Care 2016;4: 20–31.

17. Kelm DJ, Perrin JT, Cartin-Ceba R, et al. Fluid overload in patients with severe sepsis and septic shock treated with early-goal directed therapy is associated with increased acute need for fluid-related medical interventions and hospital death. Shock 2015;43:68–73.
18. Gamcrlidze MM, Intskirveli NA, Vardosanidze KD, et al. Vasoplegia in septic shock. Georgian Med News 2015;239:56–62.
19. Sharawy N. Vasoplegia in septic shock: do we fight the real enemy? J Crit Care 2014;20(1):83–7.
20. Myburgh JA, Mythen MG. Resuscitation fluids. N Engl J Med 2013;369:1243–51.
21. Weinbaum S, Tarbell JM, Damiano ER. The structure and function of the endothelial glycocalyx layer. Annu Rev Biomed Eng 2007;9:121–67.
22. Woodcock TE, Woodcock TM. Revised Starling equation and the glycocalyx model of transvascular fluid exchange: an improved paradigm for prescribing intravenous fluid therapy. Br J Anaesth 2012;108:384–94.
23. Collins SR, Blank RS, Deathrage LS, et al. The endothelial glycocalyx: emerging concepts in pulmonary edema and acute lung injury. Anesth Analg 2013;117: 664–74.
24. Lewins R. Injection of saline solutions in extraordinary quantities into the veins in cases of malignant cholera. Lancet 1832;18:243–4.
25. Frazee E, Kasahni K. Fluid management for critically ill patients: a review of the current state of fluid therapy in the intensive care unit. Kidney Dis (Basel) 2016; 2:64–71.
26. Yunos NM, Bellomo R, Story D, et al. Bench-to-bedside review: chloride in critical illness. Crit Care 2010;14:226.
27. Chowdhury AH, Cox EF, Francis ST, et al. A randomized, controlled, double-blind crossover study on the effects of 2-L infusions of 0.9% saline and Plasma-Lyte 148 on renal blood flow velocity and renal cortical tissue perfusion in healthy volunteers. Ann Surg 2012;256:18–24.
28. Shaw AD, Bagshaw SM, Goldstein SL, et al. Major complications, mortality and resource utilization after open abdominal surgery: 0.9% saline compared to Plasma-Lyte. Ann Surg 2012;255:821–9.
29. Raghunathan K, Shaw A, Nathanson B, et al. Association between the choice of IV crystalloid and in-hospital mortality among critically ill adults with sepsis. Crit Care Med 2014;42:1585–91.
30. Caironi P, Tognoni G, Masson S, et al, for the ALBIOS Study Investigators. Albumin replacement in patients with severe sepsis or septic shock. N Engl J Med 2014;370:1412–21.
31. Myburg JA, Finfer S, Bellomo R, et al, CHEST Investigators, Australian and New Zealand Intensive Care Society Clinical Trials Group. Hydroxyethyl starch or saline for fluid resuscitation in intensive care. N Engl J Med 2012;367:1901–11.
32. Boldt J. Use of albumin: an update. Br J Anaesth 2010;104:276–84.
33. Finfer S, Bellomo R, Boyce N, et al, SAFE Study Investigators. A comparison of albumin and saline for fluid resuscitation in the intensive care unit. N Eng J Med 2004;350:2247–56.
34. Myburgh J, Cooper DJ, Finfer S, et al. Saline or albumin for fluid resuscitation in patients with traumatic brain injury. N Engl J Med 2007;357:874–84.
35. Perner A, Haase N, Guttormsen AB, et al. Hydroxyethyl starch 130/0.42 versus ringer's acetate in severe sepsis. N Engl J Med 2012;367:124–34.

Does Fluid Type and Amount Affect Kidney Function in Critical Illness?

Neil J. Glassford, MBChB, PhD, MRCP(UK), AAAHMS[a,b],
Rinaldo Bellomo, MD, FRACP, FCICM, FAAHMS[a,b,c],*

KEYWORDS

- Colloid • Crystalloid • Intravenous fluid therapy • Acute kidney injury • Albumin
- Hydroxyethyl starch • Succinylated gelatin • Balanced solution

KEY POINTS

- Urine output and serum creatinine are imperfect measures of renal function, so fluid therapy given in response to these variables is likely to be of variable efficacy.
- Intravenous fluid administration can contribute to adverse renal and patient outcomes via fluid accumulation and renal edema, or direct mechanisms of toxicity.
- There is an emerging evidence base to support the preferential use of balanced crystalloid solutions in the critically ill, although the evidence for improved outcomes is largely observational to date.
- Albumin solutions have been shown to be safe in the critically ill, whereas artificial colloid solutions have been associated with adverse renal events and even increased mortality in critically ill patients.

INTRODUCTION

Intravenous fluid administration is often the initial intervention used by clinicians when faced with acute episodes of oliguria and developing acute kidney injury (AKI)[1–5]. The physiologic effects of fluid therapy tend to be brief,[6,7] and, given the range of intravenous fluids available for use and the diverse pathophysiologic states comprising critical illness, there is a risk of potentiating or exacerbating renal injury by choosing the wrong volume of the wrong fluid at the wrong time or in the wrong situation. However, the administration of fluid should not be an automatic action but a carefully considered prescription.

[a] Department of Intensive Care, Austin Hospital, 145 Studley Road, Heidelberg, Melbourne, VIC 3084, Australia; [b] Department of Epidemiology and Preventive Medicine, Monash University, Australian and New Zealand Intensive Care Research Centre, 99 Commercial Road, Melbourne, VIC 3004, Australia; [c] School of Medicine, The University of Melbourne, Grattan Street and Royal Parade, Melbourne, VIC 3010, Australia
* Corresponding author. School of Medicine, The University of Melbourne, Grattan Street and Royal Parade, Melbourne, VIC 3010, Australia.
E-mail address: Rinaldo.bellomo@austin.org.au

Crit Care Clin 34 (2018) 279–298
https://doi.org/10.1016/j.ccc.2017.12.006
0749-0704/18/© 2017 Elsevier Inc. All rights reserved.
criticalcare.theclinics.com

MEASURING RENAL DYSFUNCTION IN CRITICAL ILLNESS

Understanding the relationship between fluid administration and renal dysfunction in critical illness first requires an understanding of the currently globally accepted clinical measures of excretory renal function and their relationship to that evolving functional or structural dysfunction. The 2 most commonly used tools to diagnose renal dysfunction, both used in modern classifications of AKI, are serum creatinine concentration (sCr) and urine output (UO).

Modern definitions of AKI acknowledge the limitations of sCr in periods of acute illness. Creatinine is generated and excreted at a constant rate in health, but critical illness can result in a significant reduction in production, and its half-life can increase 6-fold to 18-fold as glomerular filtration rate (GFR) decreases.[8–11] Drugs such as ranitidine and trimethoprim interfere with tubular creatinine secretion. Jaffe-type enzymatic assays for measuring creatinine in blood can be rendered inaccurate by the presence of high concentrations of bilirubin.

An understanding of baseline renal function is also important. An sCr increase of 0.3 mg/dL in an individual with normal renal function is likely to indicate a significant reduction in underlying GFR. In individuals with chronic kidney disease, 0.2 to 0.4 mg/dL variations in serum creatinine level may represent acceptable fluctuations to a baseline of 3 to 3.5 mg/dL, and may not reflect a significant further loss of function.[12]

To add further complexity, the trajectory of the increased sCr level differs according to baseline renal function, and the severity of AKI.[13] At the least, individual variations in creatinine generation, renal reserve, the presence of liver or muscle disease, pregnancy, the volume of distribution of creatinine, and dynamic changes in the equilibrium with time need to be considered when interpreting changes in sCr level.[13,14] It can be difficult relating increasing sCr level to potential precipitants, because such events may have occurred 24 or 48 hours previously, before intensive care unit (ICU) or even hospital admission.

In addition, fluid administration, such as cardioplegia and circuit priming fluid during cardiopulmonary bypass,[15–17] or fluid overload, such as that experienced by critically ill patients in the ICU,[8,18] can dilute sCr by increasing total body water. This possibility implies that, at least in certain patients, rather than preventing or ameliorating the impact of AKI, the administration of fluid merely masks the severity of illness. It may also lead to an increased duration of exposure to a positive fluid balance and fluid overload by delaying initiation of continuous renal replacement therapy (CRRT).

HOW USEFUL IS URINE OUTPUT?

UO is an attractive marker of renal function in that it offers an apparent real-time marker of renal function, allowing the natural history of renal dysfunction to be charted. In addition, it requires no knowledge of baseline values to be calculated, unlike changes in sCr.[13,19] However, visual inspection of UO at the bedside is inaccurate. In noncatheterized patients, only intermittent volumes may be available. Data handling from the record depends on the frequency of recording. The use of diuretics, other vasoactive medications, blood products, or nephrotoxins may lead to confounding fluctuations in urine production, as may pathologic or interventional variation in hemodynamics.[19,20]

The currently extant definitions of oliguria are essentially empiric.[19,21,22] They derive from observations performed in uncontrolled small populations in the 1930s and 1940s suggesting that there is a linear reduction in GFR at absolute urinary flow rates less than approximately 0.5 mL/min (or 30 mL/h). Such rates are thought to represent the maximal concentrating ability of the kidney.[23–25] However, these were established in water deprivation studies, and the relationship between UO in early or established critical illness is less clear.

Logically, oliguria is most likely to be related to the reason for ICU admission early in that admission, whereas oliguria developing later may be a result of complications or a side effect of therapy.[26] Oliguria may be an appropriate physiologic attempt to conserve salt and water when there is increased sympathetic tone, stimulation of the renin-angiotensin-aldosterone axis, and antidiuretic hormone release as part of the response to critical illness.

The exact transition from physiologic oliguria to pathologic oliguria is uncertain and is likely to vary depending on the population being examined.[27] Transient oliguria, in which UO decreases to less than the intensity threshold levels for 1 or more hours at a time but returns to normal levels before duration threshold levels are reached, is frequently observed but is of uncertain significance in many cases. Current definitions of AKI require low UO to be present for greater than or equal to 6 hours for classification; this has been shown to be a period optimally associated with the need for subsequent dialysis, mortality, and AKI in the undifferentiated critically ill population.[28] A subset of episodes of persistent oliguria may be reversible by the restoration of renal perfusion pressure by optimizing intravascular volume status, or via other means, such as administration of a vasopressor. Although there are no well-validated methods to prospectively differentiate such episodes from periods of persistent oliguria, some clinicians advocate the use of diuretics as a stress test to identify patients with early AKI from those with transient or physiologic oliguria.[29]

Even if these individual episodes of transient and reversible oliguria are not individually associated with increased risk of subsequent AKI or mortality, then, similarly to any multihit hypothesis, the accumulation of such episodes may be important. Ongoing awareness of the burden of oliguria may allow earlier identification of patients at risk of subsequent AKI, need for CRRT, or death.

These difficulties have led to a subset of the critical care AKI literature presenting only data on renal dysfunction as diagnosed by changes in sCr. Recent studies have shown that oliguria is associated with mortality independently of the development of creatinine-defined AKI.[30] Despite this association, none of the modern classifications of AKI or oliguria are incorporated into modern illness severity scoring systems.[31–34] In addition, many studies fail to account or correct for the effect of a positive fluid balance on serum creatinine or other biomarker concentrations when diagnosing AKI. Making such corrections has been shown to identify AKI earlier, with patients identified as having AKI postcorrection having similar outcomes to those whose AKI status is independent of fluid balance.

Peptide and other chemical biomarkers, such as neutrophil gelatinase-associated lipocalin,[35,36] cell-cycle arrest biomarkers,[37] and endostatin,[38,39] have been mooted as being useful for predicting the significance of periods of oliguria, or the development of subsequent AKI, or for diagnosing the presence of established AKI. Predictive biomarkers would be useful and would allow efforts to be focused on patients in whom intervention may be beneficial at a point at which progression may be halted or severity may be ameliorated. However, beyond oliguria, which may not be pathologic, there are no other immediately evident clinical signs of renal distress, and so the ability to characterize the natural history of such biomarkers and calibrate them depending on the position of the patient in their clinical course is limited in the undifferentiated critical care population.[28]

Fluid therapy may be initiated or modified in response to either trigger, although fluid bolus therapy (FBT) administration as a response to oliguria is better represented in the literature. The administration of fluid to patients potentially losing the ability to regulate their fluid and electrolyte balance can contribute to AKI and patient outcome in 2 main ways: via the effects of fluid accumulation, or the physicochemical and pharmacologic effects of the fluids themselves.

ARE FLUIDS A REQUIRED COMPONENT OF RENAL RESUSCITATION?

The traditional paradigm of AKI management often involves aggressive fluid resuscitation, or at least the maintenance of euvolemia. Oliguria has been shown in both regional and international studies to be a frequent trigger for subsequent FBT, and subsequent change in UO is often used as a measure of response to therapy,[1,3] even though these values in reality may be markedly divorced from clinician expectation.[4] Fluid responsiveness is a complex topic, and outside of the scope of this article, but it is worth noting that, in a recent prospective cross-sectional study, more than 40% of fluid challenges were given without reference to variables predicting fluid responsiveness.[3] Moreover, current academic definitions of fluid responsiveness revolve around changes in stroke volume or cardiac output, but most clinicians define the success of a response based on changes in mean arterial blood pressure.[3,40]

A recent prospective cross-sectional study on the epidemiology of AKI in 33 countries suggests sepsis to be the most common cause for AKI in the critically ill, followed by hypovolemia, drugs, and cardiogenic shock. Although the mechanism by which fluid status was determined was not reported, hypovolemia was only thought to contribute in 34% of cases.[41] In these cases, the classic physiologic paradigm of restoration of GFR and renal oxygen supply by increasing preload, stroke volume, cardiac output, and hence renal blood flow seems logical. At least, it would if the likely distribution and dissipation kinetics of the fluid between conduit and capacitance circulations could be identified, or even if reliable predictors of fluid responsiveness were available, given the potential for harm associated with fluid accumulation in the critically ill, specifically those with AKI.[42,43]

In septic AKI, a complex pathophysiologic state of variable or even increased renal blood flow, microvascular abnormalities, glycocalyceal disruption and endothelial leak, direct inflammatory injury, increased oxidative stress and tubule dysfunction, and subsequent organ dysfunction, it is difficult to identify an obvious therapeutic role for fluid therapy.[44] The administration of fluid to oliguric patients at risk of AKI has an obvious consequence: fluid accumulation. The consequences of solute accumulation and exposure are discussed later, but the consequences of an increasingly positive fluid balance, particularly among patients with AKI, have been well documented (**Table 1**). In healthy volunteers given 2000-mL crystalloid infusions over 60 minutes, significant increases in renal volume secondary to increased interstitial edema were observed.[45] As an encapsulated organ, increased tissue volume leads to increased resistance to venous return, with subsequent reductions in GFR; such a relationship evolves exponentially on maximizing the distensibility of the capsule. In severe cases, given the often-precarious perfusion of the renal medulla, this may contribute to renal ischemia.[46–50] This increased renal venous pressure may be reflected systemically as an increased central venous pressure (CVP). Fluid administration can directly damage glycocalyceal integrity, lead to atrial natriuretic peptide release, and exacerbate interstitial edema,[51] overwhelming the ability of the lymphatic system to clear the interstitium.[52] Edema of the brain, heart, and lungs may directly or indirectly contribute to AKI by reducing renal blood flow or oxygen supply.[53,54] Although current guidelines suggest a CVP target as part of the fluid management of severe sepsis, such observations indicate that CVP may best serve as a limit for

Table 1
Key studies examining the relationships between fluid balance, acute kidney injury, and mortality

Study	Year	Design	Population	Findings
PICARD[41–43]	2004, 2009, 2010	Prospective observational	610 adult ICU patients with AKI, 253 with complete sCr data	Significant linear trend with increasing proportion of days spent in FO for increasing mortality in patients requiring RRT FA delays diagnosis
FACTT[44]	2011	Post hoc analyses of RCT	306 critically ill adult ventilated patients with AKI	FA masked AKI diagnosis; independent association between FB adjusted AKI status and mortality In patients with AKI, FB independently associated with mortality
RENAL[45]	2012	Post hoc analyses of RCT	1453 critically ill adult patients with AKI requiring RRT	Negative mean daily FB independently associated with ICU and 90-d survival
FINNAKI[23,46]	2012, 2015	Post hoc analyses of observational study	2160 adult ICU patients	FO greatest in patients with increased sCr level and oliguria FO independently associated with mortality in patients requiring RRT
Garzotto[47]	2016	Prospective observational	1734 adult ICU patients	FO independently associated with mortality in patients with or without AKI Speed of FA independently associated with mortality in patients with AKI
Neyra[48]	2016	Retrospective observational	2632 septic adult ICU patients	AKI and CKD status influence FB and FO status Independent association between FB and mortality in patients with AKI and CKD
Thongprayoon[49]	2016	Retrospective observational	7696 adult ICU patients	FA delays AKI diagnosis AKI an independent predictor of mortality when adjusted for FB sCr an improved predictor of mortality when adjusted for FB

Abbreviations: CKD, chronic kidney disease; FA, fluid accumulation; FACTT, Fluids and Catheters Treatment Trial; FB, fluid balance; FINNAKI, Finnish Acute Kidney Injury Study; FO, fluid overload; PICARD, Program to Improve Care in Acute Renal Disease; RCT, randomized controlled trial; RENAL, Randomized Evaluation of Normal versus Augmented Level Replacement Therapy Study; RRT, renal replacement therapy.

fluid resuscitation.[55] Importantly, the pilot Conservative Versus Liberal Approach to Fluid Therapy of Septic Shock in Intensive Care (CLASSIC) trial shows that attempts to restrict resuscitation volumes in patients with septic shock are feasible and may improve renal outcomes.[56] In 9 ICUs in Finland and Denmark, 151 patients with septic shock were randomized to restrictive fluid therapy (isotonic crystalloid fluid boluses of 250–500 mL for evidence of severe hypoperfusion only) or standard care (isotonic crystalloid fluid boluses for as long as hemodynamic improvement observed). Although methodologically imperfect, with some baseline differences between groups, significant differences were shown in volume of resuscitation fluid given over the ICU stay and in cumulative fluid balance at day 5. Although no mortality difference was observed, AKI was more likely to worsen in patients receiving standard care (restrictive, 37% vs standard, 54%; $P = .03$).

Cardiogenic shock, a low-output state with increased filling pressures, tissue hypoperfusion, with pulmonary and more global venous congestion, is a common cause of AKI, but is one to which fluid therapy is likely to contribute, not ameliorate. In more than 2500 patients with cardiovascular disease undergoing right heart cardiac catheterization over a 17-year period, increasing CVP was independently associated with decreasing estimated GFR, and with mortality.[57] In a cohort of 145 patients hospitalized with advanced decompensated heart failure for pulmonary artery–guided treatment, increased CVP was shown to be associated with worsening renal function.[58] Most recently, in a retrospective analysis of 9000 patients from the Medical Information Mart for Intensive Care (MIMIC) database,[59] increased CVP was shown to have an independent association with 28-day mortality in all patients, with a suggestion that this relationship was stronger in patients with AKI. Patients in the higher 2 CVP quartiles also had significantly higher median fluid balances at 72 hours.[60]

Further fluid may be received in the form of postoperative FBT.[61] In a post hoc analysis of a prospective observational trial of 282 patients undergoing cardiac surgery in a tertiary center, low perioperative mean arterial pressure and increasing fluid accumulation were shown to be independently associated with need for renal replacement therapy (RRT) and mortality.[62]

MECHANISMS OF RENAL INJURY RELATED TO TYPE OF FLUID

Independent of the effects of fluid accumulation, the type of fluid given to patients with renal dysfunction may have a significant impact on disease progression or patient outcome.[63] The contents of commonly used crystalloid and colloid solutions are presented in **Table 2**. Sodium-rich and chloride-rich solutions may trigger afferent arteriolar vasoconstriction via tubuloglomerular feedback.[64] There is a theoretic concern that the transient increases in plasma oncotic pressure observed on administration of colloid solutions reduces the net filtration pressure across the glomerular filtration barrier, leading to a reduction in GFR, although such concerns do not seem to be borne out in clinical practice.[65–67] Synthetic colloids have been shown to cause osmotic nephrosis, with vacuolization, swelling, and distortion of proximal tubule cells, changes that can permanently impair renal function (**Fig. 1**).[68,69]

SODIUM, CHLORIDE, AND BALANCED SOLUTIONS

The recent Fluid – Translating Research into Practice (Fluid-TRIPS) study provided a fascinating insight into international fluid resuscitation practices, as well as trends in resuscitation over the period 2007 to 2014.[70] Over this time period, the use of crystalloids increased compared with colloids, and the use of buffered, or balanced, salt solutions increased while the use of saline decreased. Although overall colloid use

Table 2
Constituents, pH, and osmolality of commonly used intravenous fluids, with normal plasma values for comparison

Fluid Class		Intravenous Fluids							
		Colloids					Crystalloids		
			Hydroxyethyl Starch						
Fluid Type	Plasma[a]	Gelatin	Voluven	Volulyte	Albumin 4%	Albumin 20%	0.9% Saline Solution	Hartmann Solution	Plasma-Lyte 148
Brand Name		Gelofusine							
Substitution/MW	—	30	130/0.4	130/0.4	—	—	—	—	—
pH	7.35–7.45	7.1–7.7	4–5.5	5.7–6.5	6.7–7.3	6.7–7.3	4.5–7	5–7	4–6.5
Na (mmol/L)	135–145	154	154	137	140	40–100	154	130	140
K (mmol/L)	3.5–5.2	—	—	4	—	—	—	4	5
Ca (mmol/L)	2.1–2.6	—	—	—	—	—	—	3	—
Mg (mmol/L)	0.7–1.1	—	—	—	—	—	—	—	1.5
Cl (mmol/L)	95–110	120	154	110	128	19	154	110	98
Lactate (mmol/L)	0.5–1	—	—	—	—	—	—	28	—
Albumin (g/L)	35–55	—	—	—	40	40	—	—	—
Octanoate (mmol/L)	—	—	—	—	6.4	32	—	—	—
Acetate (mmol/L)	—	—	—	—	—	—	—	—	27
Gluconate (mmol/L)	—	—	—	—	—	—	—	—	23
Osmolality (mOsm/kg H$_2$O)	285–295	274	308	286.5	250	130	308	275	295

Abbreviation: MW, molecular weight.
[a] Normal ranges for human plasma values.

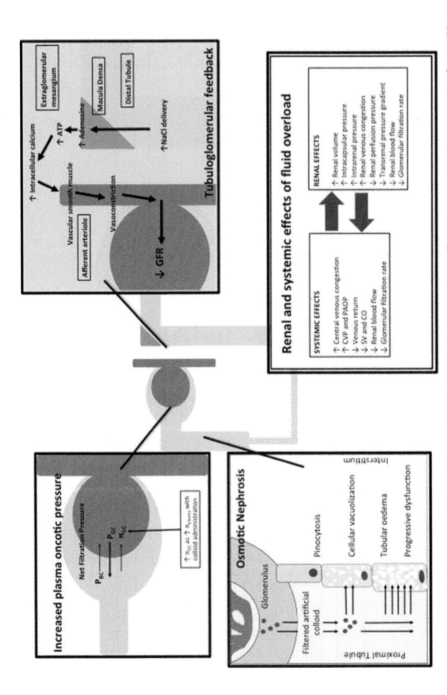

Fig. 1. Pathophysiology of fluid administration in AKI. π_{GC} oncotic pressure in glomerular capillaries; π_{plasma} oncotic pressure in plasma; CO, cardiac output; CVP, central venous pressure; GFR, glomerular filtration rate; PAOP, pulmonary artery occlusion pressure; P_{BC} hydrostatic pressure in Bowman capsule; P_{GC} hydrostatic pressure in glomerular capillaries; SV, stroke volume.

decreased, albumin use increased, indicating a significant decrease in the use of artificial colloids, although there was significant geographic variation in the use of colloid solutions. On univariate analysis, no significant association was shown between the presence of oliguria or significant renal impairment (defined as a sCr $\geq$170 μmol/L), and subsequent choice of fluid type. However, after multivariable analysis, patients already requiring RRT were shown to be more likely to be resuscitated with colloids and less likely with crystalloids compared with those not requiring such support.

This increased use of crystalloid solutions, and emerging preference for balanced solutions, has been shown in observational studies,[3,71] in surveys of physician preference,[4] and in regional examinations of fluid sales data.[72] Sodium-rich fluids are frequently administered in the ICU, leading to a positive sodium balance and hypernatremia, and possibly contributing to respiratory dysfunction, AKI, and mortality.[73–76] Moreover, sodium administration is often linked to chloride administration, and observational evidence has linked chloride loading with AKI and possibly mortality.[77–79]

A multicenter, cluster-randomized, double-crossover, randomized controlled trial (RCT) comparing balanced and unbalanced crystalloids showed no mortality advantage on an undifferentiated population of critically ill patients (n = 2278), or on subgroup analysis of those with sepsis (n = 84).[80] There were no differences between groups in incidence of risk, injury, failure, loss, end-stage (RIFLE) or kidney disease: improving global outcomes (KDIGO) stage AKI, or RRT use or indications for initiation between groups. However, the wide confidence intervals around the point estimate of the treatment effect in a heterogeneous population with a low incidence of AKI, and the low number of clusters in the trial design, preclude an effect on renal function from being ruled out.[81,82]

In a prospective, open-label, cluster-randomized, multiple-crossover trial comparing the use of saline and balanced crystalloids in a single medical ICU where the type of fluid administered alternated monthly after random allocation, no difference was seen between groups in the rate of major adverse kidney events at 30 days (MAKE30), need for RRT, or incidence of KDIGO stage 2 AKI or greater, in the cohort (n = 974). On subgroup analysis of the 260 patients with sepsis or septic shock, a significant reduction in the risk of the composite MAKE30 outcome was reported with the use of balanced solutions (OR, 0.56; 95% confidence interval [CI], 0.33–0.94). However, the study was not powered to analyze this outcome, and the brief turnover period of the intervention means that patients present in the unit during crossover were exposed to both fluids.[83] Both of these studies were planned as pilot investigations for larger, potentially definitive interventions. There is even limited evidence that substitution of balanced solutions may result in net health care cost savings.[84]

Evidence seems to be emerging that the use of balanced solutions may be preferable to chloride-rich alternatives; such solutions should be used in AKI with caution. Further information will be provided by studies already underway or nearing completion. The Isotonic Solutions and Major Adverse Renal Events Trial (SMART) is a pragmatic cluster-randomized, multiple crossover trial, intended to recruit 14,000 patients, to compare rates of the MAKE30 composite outcome between patients randomized to saline or balanced crystalloid solutions.[85] The Plasma-Lyte 148 Versus Saline (PLUS) study, intending to recruit almost 9000 patients from 50 Australian and New Zealand ICUs to compare 90-day mortality and a variety of renal and other patient-centered outcomes in patients randomized to either buffered crystalloid solution or saline, may provide a more definitive answer in the near future.[86]

ALBUMIN SOLUTIONS

Serum albumin is an essential plasma protein, and hypoalbuminemia is common in critical illness. Albumin has a variety of homeostatic and predictive roles in health and disease, and human albumin solution has been administered clinically for more than 5 decades. Albumin has been shown to be as safe as saline when given for the purposes of volume expansion or fluid resuscitation to an undifferentiated critically ill population. The Saline Versus Albumin Fluid Evaluation (SAFE) Study randomized 6997 patients from 16 ICUs to intravascular volume expansion with either 4% albumin or normal saline. There were no reported differences in need for mechanical ventilation, RRT, length of hospital or ICU stay, or 28-day all-cause mortality.[87] This was the first large, well-conducted RCT to show the safety of albumin solutions in the heterogeneous population of the ICU after decades of controversy.[88] However, it was neither designed nor powered to show superiority to saline in different groups of critically ill patients, nor to explore renal outcomes. A non–statistically significantly increased risk of mortality with albumin administration in patients with trauma, and a similarly non–statistically significant reduction in mortality in patients with severe sepsis, were observed in the trial, resulting in the publication of important subgroup analyses.[89,90]

In a post hoc analysis of 460 SAFE patients with radiological evidence of brain injury, a history of head trauma, and a Glasgow Coma Scale score of less than or equal to 13, 231 received albumin and the remainder saline when resuscitation was required. There was a significantly greater risk of death at 24 months in patients treated with albumin, despite similar baseline characteristics (relative risk [RR], 1.63; 95% CI, 1.17–2.26; $P = .003$). In the approximately two-thirds of each group with severe brain injury (GCS ≤ 8), the risk of death was greater (RR, 1.88; 95% CI, 1.31–2.70; $P<.001$). Serum albumin level was higher in the albumin group on all 4 days, and their net fluid balance was greater on the first 2 study days, compared with the saline group. This finding seemed to be driven by volume of study fluid delivered. In addition, the CVP of the albumin group was approximately 1 mm Hg higher over the first 2 study days.[89] No renal outcomes were reported in this analysis or on a subsequent post hoc analysis using complex pattern mixture modeling to suggest increased ICP over the first 7 days of ICU admission as the cause of the observed excess mortality.[91]

Given the suggestion of a mortality advantage when resuscitating patients with severe sepsis with albumin compared with saline, a subgroup analysis of 1218 patients was undertaken. There were no significant demographic differences between groups at baseline, but those patients receiving albumin were given significantly less study fluid over the first 3 days of the study, with no differences in transfusion requirements, vasopressor use, or need for mechanical ventilation. They also received significantly less fluid overall over the first 2 days.[90] There was no significant difference between groups in the proportion of patients requiring RRT, or in the renal component of the Sequential Organ Failure Assessment (SOFA) score over the first 7 days of inclusion. No information regarding modern definitions of AKI were available; SAFE was published the same year as the Acute Dialysis Quality Initiative (ADQI) RIFLE definitions.[19] In the 76% of patients with sufficient information, an independent association between albumin administration and survival was shown following adjustment for illness severity, gender, age, postoperative admission, source of sepsis, and serum albumin level, with a reduction in the odds ratio (OR) for death at 28 days (OR, 0.71; 95% CI, 0.52–0.97; $P = .03$).[90]

The largest trial to date comparing the efficacy of albumin with saline resuscitation in sepsis was performed in critically ill children in sub-Saharan Africa.[92] A 2-stratum, multicenter, open, randomized controlled study, the Fluid Expansion as Supportive Therapy (FEAST) trial, compared the effects of albumin or saline resuscitation with maintenance therapy only on mortality in more than 3000 children with clinical evidence of impaired perfusion. The details and importance of these findings have been dissected and discussed elsewhere, but essentially no differences were found in primary or secondary end points including 48-hour or 4-week mortality between the albumin and saline groups.[92–98] The most provocative findings of the FEAST trial relate to the comparison of FBT with no resuscitation. In this population, the absolute risk of death in children with suspected severe infection was increased by 3.3% by FBT with albumin or saline (RR, 1.45; 95% CI, 1.13–1.86; $P = .003$), with most occurring within 48 hours. No heterogeneity was found between centers or across age groups, and the difference persisted across all prespecified subgroups.[92,97] Given the pragmatic nature and resource-poor setting of the study, limited information regarding renal function is available. However, the incidence of severe acid-base disturbances (pH <7.2, base deficit ≥ 8 mmol/L) or hyperkalemia (potassium level >6.5 mmol/L) was the same in all 3 groups, implying a similar degree of biochemical disarray, possibly secondary to AKI.[97]

A single-center, retrospective observational study investigated the impact of the volume and type of fluid administered over the first 36 postoperative hours on development of AKI over the first 4 postoperative days in 984 patients at risk of cardiac surgery–associated AKI following cardiopulmonary bypass.[99] A dose-dependent risk of RIFLE AKI was observed with the use of albumin or pentastarch 10% solutions. Although attempts were made to propensity match and a case-control analysis was performed, the study was unpowered for such post hoc analyses. Fluid balance was included in the modeling attempts, but sCr diagnosis of RIFLE AKI category was not corrected for fluid accumulation, and patients receiving albumin had significantly lower fluid balances over the first 36 hours of the study. Overall, it is likely that receipt of albumin administration was an unconscious marker of illness severity. Moreover, it is impossible to identify whether surgical or anesthetic team fluid preference, considered alone or as part of the larger question of the overall team performance, acts as a systematic confounder.[100] Given the lack of a representative variable, even the use of a propensity score would not take this into account. It does highlight the complexities of research in the fluid space and the need for specific research questions in specific populations.[42]

These studies were performed with near iso-oncotic 4% to 5% albumin solutions; hyperoncotic 20% to 25% solutions are also available. Hyperoncotic albumin solutions have been associated with adverse renal events, although the most compelling evidence supporting this relationship comes from a large, prospective observational study in shocked ICU patients requiring fluid resuscitation. Hyperoncotic albumin was associated with an increased risk of renal event or ICU death. Although it included more than 1000 patients, the study did not use a modern definition of AKI and failed to account for the effect of fluid status on diagnosis. Despite propensity analysis, there were key differences between patients indicating a significantly greater degree of critical illness, including higher baseline levels of organ support and greater degree of organ dysfunction in those receiving hyperoncotic solutions, and these are unlikely to be fully accounted for by the adjusted analysis.[101]

This finding is consistent with the findings of a retrospective single center study comparing the hemodynamic effects of FBT with 4% and 20% albumin solutions in 202 critically ill patients. ICU mortality was significantly higher in those receiving 20% albumin, although patients receiving 20% albumin had significantly higher APACHE III (Acute Physiology and Chronic Health Evaluation) scores and differing distributions of comorbidities, as well as a significantly greater incidence of ICU mortality. This difference disappeared after adjustment for illness severity. Despite being given to more severely ill patients, the hemodynamic effects of 20% albumin FBT were similar to those of 4%. Although UO and AKI outcomes were not reported, significantly smaller quantities of fluid, sodium, and chloride were delivered.[102]

Two large RCTs have explored albumin supplementation in the critically ill, with 20% albumin being given routinely[66] or to maintain a target serum albumin concentration.[65] Only 1 trial, the Albumin Italian Outcome in Sepsis (ALBIOS) study, has been published in its entirety.[65] Neither study showed any mortality or renal advantage following albumin supplementation. However, in the ALBIOS study, rates of AKI used the RIFLE rather than the more sensitive AKI network criteria, and failed to account for the significant difference in fluid balance between groups, which may have been masking higher rates of AKI in the control group.[65] Given the absence of a difference in rates of RRT or morality, the potential significance of this remains questionable.

Albumin solutions encapsulate the discussions regarding ideal electrolyte composition and osmolality of resuscitation fluids relative to plasma. Given that 20% and 4% albumin seem equally hemodynamically efficacious and that their administration has been proved in the undifferentiated critically ill population to be as safe as saline administration, they offer a unique research opportunity to assess the effects of chloride and sodium loads and osmolality on the critically ill. However, the cost of these solutions in many jurisdictions would hinder investigations on the scale required to observe differences in mortality, or even appropriate secondary outcomes.

HYDROXYETHYL STARCH

It would now be difficult to recommend or condone the use of intravenous hydroxyethyl starch (HES) solutions in critically ill patients, particularly those with AKI, sepsis, or burns. Derived from maize or potato, these modified polysaccharides are degraded in plasma and filtered by the kidney, although other tissues take up a substantial portion of circulating HES. This finding can be shown at necroscopy, often a considerable period of time after administration.

There is evidence of a dose-dependent effect of HES administration on AKI and need for RRT, and its use conveys no mortality advantage, either in these studies[103,104] or on systematic review.[105-107] Several international agencies banned or placed heavy restrictions on their use following the publication of these studies. However, manufacturers of the products appealed, and questions were raised regarding the analysis and interpretation of the largest of these studies, the Crystalloid versus Hydroxyethyl Starch Trial.[108-110] Given the concerns regarding the results of the study, and the potential implications of any unidentified errors, the trial sponsors commissioned an independent reanalysis of the data using the material by the highly regarded Duke Clinical Research Institute. No substantial differences were identified between analyses, and certainly none affecting the conclusions of the study.[111] Although an unusual step, this represents a new standard of excellence in methodological rigor and transparency of reporting. Moving forward, independent concurrent analysis may be considered an essential component of trial design in sensitive or controversial areas.

GELATIN SOLUTIONS

Derived from bovine collagen and available in different markets in different formulations, recent interest in gelatin solutions has been rekindled,[112,113] possibly as the availability of HES has dwindled. However, many of the features making HES unsuitable as a resuscitation fluid apply similarly to gelatins.[114] In a rat model of septic shock, animals treated with gelatin or starch solution showed peritubular capillary dilatation, detachment of basement membrane epithelial cells, increased tubular vacuolation, and increased cell death at necroscopy. Specific to animals given gelatin solution was increased interstitial edema and loss of the proximal tubular cell brush border. Serum urea and sCr were also significantly higher in animals from the gelatin group compared with sham-treated animals. Some of these findings were more significant than in animals given starch.[68]

In Australian and New Zealand ICUs, gelatin use has significantly decreased since 2007.[71,72] Internationally, a recent survey indicated that approximately a third of intensivists thought gelatin solutions were acceptable for use as a resuscitation fluid, although the proportion varied significantly between jurisdictions.[4] Certain gelatin solutions inhibit platelet aggregation, and they seem to cause a more profound inhibition of von Willebrand factor and factor VIII than modern HES solutions. These effects on coagulation resulted in a removal from the market in the United States for some formulations almost 40 years ago.[115–117] For example, patients undergoing cardiac surgery required significantly more platelet transfusions and those with sepsis required more red cell and fresh frozen plasma transfusions when treated with gelatins or HES than when treated with crystalloids, in 2 large, well-conducted, observational studies. These same studies showed a higher rate of AKI and greater need for RRT in patients treated with gelatins compared with crystalloids, with no quicker resolution in shock.[118,119] Moreover, in cardiac surgical patients, following extensive appropriate adjustment and propensity score stratification, the odds of in-hospital mortality were increased (post–propensity stratification OR, 1.40; 95% CI, 1.07–1.84; $P = .016$).

A recent systematic review summarized the randomized, observational, and animal data on gelatin use in the critically ill. The gross clinical and methodological heterogeneity of the identified studies should have precluded attempts to provide pooled estimates of effect, and the confidence intervals for mortality, transfusion, and AKI were wide and included unity. However, even with these methodological issues, a strong signal of increased risk of anaphylaxis compared with crystalloid solutions was observed across these data (RR, 3.01; 95% CI, 1.27–7.14).[120] No other high-quality investigations have shown a mortality advantage with gelatin administration.[121] Given the risks associated with artificial colloid use, the fact they accumulate in tubular cells and extrarenal tissues, their cost compared with crystalloids, and the lack of a demonstrated renal or mortality advantage, it is difficult to recommend their use in the modern management of AKI.

SUMMARY

Fluid administration should not be an automatic prescriptive reaction to oliguria or increasing creatinine level in the critically ill. Fluid accumulation is hazardous and has a complex relationship with oliguria, AKI, and mortality. Artificial colloids seem to be universally injurious in patients with renal dysfunction. Crystalloid and albumin solutions seem to be safe, but albumin has not been shown to offer any renal advantage. Although an evolving physician preference for balanced solutions is clear, RCTs have yet to show a convincing renal or mortality advantage. Until large, well-designed trials provide clear guidance regarding the optimal fluid choices to prevent or ameliorate AKI, or promote renal recovery, all care should be taken to avoid further harm in this vulnerable population.

REFERENCES

1. Bihari S, Prakash S, Bersten AD. Post resuscitation fluid boluses in severe sepsis or septic shock: prevalence and efficacy (price study). Shock 2013; 40(1):28–34.
2. Boulain T, Boisrame-Helms J, Ehrmann S, et al. Volume expansion in the first 4 days of shock: a prospective multicentre study in 19 French intensive care units. Intensive Care Med 2015;41(2):248–56.
3. Cecconi M, Hofer C, Teboul JL, et al. Fluid challenges in intensive care: the FENICE study: a global inception cohort study. Intensive Care Med 2015; 41(9):1529–37.
4. Glassford NJ, Martensson J, Eastwood GM, et al. Defining the characteristics and expectations of fluid bolus therapy: a worldwide perspective. J Crit Care 2016;35:126–32.
5. Prowle JR, Liu YL, Licari E, et al. Oliguria as predictive biomarker of acute kidney injury in critically ill patients. Crit Care 2011;15(4):R172.
6. Lipcsey M, Chiong J, Subiakto I, et al. Primary fluid bolus therapy for infection-associated hypotension in the emergency department. Crit Care Resusc 2015; 17(1):6–11.
7. Lipcsey M, Subiakto I, Chiong J, et al. Epidemiology of secondary fluid bolus therapy for infection-associated hypotension. Crit Care Resusc 2016;18(3): 165–73.
8. Liu KD, Thompson BT, Ancukiewicz M, et al. Acute kidney injury in patients with acute lung injury: impact of fluid accumulation on classification of acute kidney injury and associated outcomes. Crit Care Med 2011;39(12):2665–71.
9. Doi K, Yuen PS, Eisner C, et al. Reduced production of creatinine limits its use as marker of kidney injury in sepsis. J Am Soc Nephrol 2009;20(6):1217–21.
10. Thomas ME, Blaine C, Dawnay A, et al. The definition of acute kidney injury and its use in practice. Kidney Int 2015;87(1):62–73.
11. Clark WR, Mueller BA, Kraus MA, et al. Quantification of creatinine kinetic parameters in patients with acute renal failure. Kidney Int 1998;54(2):554–60.
12. Palevsky PM, Liu KD, Brophy PD, et al. KDOQI US commentary on the 2012 KDIGO clinical practice guideline for acute kidney injury. Am J Kidney Dis 2013;61(5):649–72.
13. Waikar SS, Bonventre JV. Creatinine kinetics and the definition of acute kidney injury. J Am Soc Nephrol 2009;20(3):672–9.
14. Ostermann M, Joannidis M. Acute kidney injury 2016: diagnosis and diagnostic workup. Crit Care 2016;20(1):299.
15. Ho J, Reslerova M, Gali B, et al. Serum creatinine measurement immediately after cardiac surgery and prediction of acute kidney injury. Am J Kidney Dis 2012; 59(2):196–201.
16. Grynberg K, Polkinghorne KR, Ford S, et al. Early serum creatinine accurately predicts acute kidney injury post cardiac surgery. BMC Nephrol 2017;18(1):93.
17. Moore E, Tobin A, Reid D, et al. The impact of fluid balance on the detection, classification and outcome of acute kidney injury after cardiac surgery. J Cardiothorac Vasc Anesth 2015;29(5):1229–35.
18. Macedo E, Bouchard J, Soroko SH, et al. Fluid accumulation, recognition and staging of acute kidney injury in critically-ill patients. Crit Care 2010;14(3):R82.
19. Bellomo R, Ronco C, Kellum JA, et al, Acute Dialysis Quality Initiative Workgroup. Acute renal failure – definition, outcome measures, animal models, fluid therapy and information technology needs: the Second International Consensus

Conference of the Acute Dialysis Quality Initiative (ADQI) Group. Crit Care 2004; 8(4):R204–12.

20. Legrand M, Payen D. Understanding urine output in critically ill patients. Ann Intensive Care 2011;1(1):13.

21. Kellum JA, Lameire N, KDIGO AKI Guideline Work Group. Diagnosis, evaluation, and management of acute kidney injury: a KDIGO summary (Part 1). Crit Care 2013;17(1):204.

22. Mehta RL, Kellum JA, Shah SV, et al. Acute Kidney Injury Network: report of an initiative to improve outcomes in acute kidney injury. Crit Care 2007;11(2):R31.

23. Chasis H, Smith HW. The excretion of urea in normal man and in subjects with glomerulonephritis. J Clin Invest 1938;17(3):347–58.

24. Chesley LC. Renal excretion at low urine volumes and the mechanism of oliguria. J Clin Invest 1938;17(5):591–7.

25. Gamble JL. The Harvey Lectures, Series XLIII, 1946-1947: physiological information gained from studies on the life raft ration. Nutr Rev 1989;47(7):199–201.

26. Mandelbaum T, Lee J, Scott DJ, et al. Empirical relationships among oliguria, creatinine, mortality, and renal replacement therapy in the critically ill. Intensive Care Med 2013;39(3):414–9.

27. Vaara ST, Parviainen I, Pettila V, et al. Association of oliguria with the development of acute kidney injury in the critically ill. Kidney Int 2016;89(1):200–8.

28. Md Ralib A, Pickering JW, Shaw GM, et al. The urine output definition of acute kidney injury is too liberal. Crit Care 2013;17(3):R112.

29. Koyner JL, Davison DL, Brasha-Mitchell E, et al. Furosemide stress test and biomarkers for the prediction of AKI severity. J Am Soc Nephrol 2015;26(8): 2023–31.

30. Kellum JA, Sileanu FE, Murugan R, et al. Classifying AKI by urine output versus serum creatinine level. J Am Soc Nephrol 2015;26(9):2231–8.

31. Higgins TL, Teres D, Copes WS, et al. Assessing contemporary intensive care unit outcome: an updated Mortality Probability Admission Model (MPM0-III). Crit Care Med 2007;35(3):827–35.

32. Knaus WA, Wagner DP, Draper EA, et al. The APACHE III prognostic system. Risk prediction of hospital mortality for critically ill hospitalized adults. Chest 1991;100(6):1619–36.

33. Metnitz PG, Moreno RP, Almeida E, et al. SAPS 3–From evaluation of the patient to evaluation of the intensive care unit. Part 1: objectives, methods and cohort description. Intensive Care Med 2005;31(10):1336–44.

34. Moreno RP, Metnitz PG, Almeida E, et al. SAPS 3–From evaluation of the patient to evaluation of the intensive care unit. Part 2: development of a prognostic model for hospital mortality at ICU admission. Intensive Care Med 2005; 31(10):1345–55.

35. Martensson J, Glassford NJ, Jones S, et al. Urinary neutrophil gelatinase-associated lipocalin to hepcidin ratio as a biomarker of acute kidney injury in intensive care unit patients. Minerva Anestesiol 2015;81(11):1192–200.

36. Martensson J, Bellomo R. The rise and fall of NGAL in acute kidney injury. Blood Purif 2014;37(4):304–10.

37. Bell M, Larsson A, Venge P, et al. Assessment of cell-cycle arrest biomarkers to predict early and delayed acute kidney injury. Dis Markers 2015;2015:158658.

38. Martensson J, Vaara ST, Pettila V, et al. Assessment of plasma endostatin to predict acute kidney injury in critically ill patients. Acta Anaesthesiol Scand 2017; 61(10):1286–95.

39. Martensson J, Jonsson N, Glassford NJ, et al. Plasma endostatin may improve acute kidney injury risk prediction in critically ill patients. Ann Intensive Care 2016;6(1):6.

40. Toscani L, Aya HD, Antonakaki D, et al. What is the impact of the fluid challenge technique on diagnosis of fluid responsiveness? A systematic review and meta-analysis. Crit Care 2017;21(1):207.

41. Hoste EA, Bagshaw SM, Bellomo R, et al. Epidemiology of acute kidney injury in critically ill patients: the multinational AKI-EPI study. Intensive Care Med 2015; 41(8):1411–23.

42. Glassford NJ, Bellomo R. The complexities of intravenous fluid research: questions of scale, volume, and accumulation. Korean J Crit Care Med 2016;31(4): 276–99.

43. Glassford NJ, Bellomo R. The role of oliguria and the absence of fluid administration and balance information in illness severity scores. Korean Journal of Critical Care Medicine 2017;32(2):106–23.

44. Bellomo R, Kellum JA, Ronco C, et al. Acute kidney injury in sepsis. Intensive Care Med 2017;43(6):816–28.

45. Chowdhury AH, Cox EF, Francis ST, et al. A randomized, controlled, double-blind crossover study on the effects of 2-L infusions of 0.9% saline and Plasma-Lyte® 148 on renal blood flow velocity and renal cortical tissue perfusion in healthy volunteers. Ann Surg 2012;256(1):18–24.

46. Boyd JH, Forbes J, Nakada TA, et al. Fluid resuscitation in septic shock: a positive fluid balance and elevated central venous pressure are associated with increased mortality. Crit Care Med 2011;39(2):259–65.

47. Legrand M, Dupuis C, Simon C, et al. Association between systemic hemodynamics and septic acute kidney injury in critically ill patients: a retrospective observational study. Crit Care 2013;17(6):R278.

48. Marik PE, Baram M, Vahid B. Does central venous pressure predict fluid responsiveness? A systematic review of the literature and the tale of seven mares. Chest 2008;134(1):172–8.

49. Wong BT, Chan MJ, Glassford NJ, et al. Mean arterial pressure and mean perfusion pressure deficit in septic acute kidney injury. J Crit Care 2015;30(5): 975–81.

50. Cruces P, Salas C, Lillo P, et al. The renal compartment: a hydraulic view. Intensive Care Med Exp 2014;2(1):26.

51. Chappell D, Bruegger D, Potzel J, et al. Hypervolemia increases release of atrial natriuretic peptide and shedding of the endothelial glycocalyx. Crit Care 2014; 18(5):538.

52. O'Connor ME, Prowle JR. Fluid overload. Crit Care Clin 2015;31(4):803–21.

53. Okusa MD. The changing pattern of acute kidney injury: from one to multiple organ failure. Contrib Nephrol 2010;165:153–8.

54. Virzi G, Day S, de Cal M, et al. Heart-kidney crosstalk and role of humoral signaling in critical illness. Crit Care 2014;18(1):201.

55. Dellinger RP, Levy MM, Rhodes A, et al. Surviving sepsis campaign: international guidelines for management of severe sepsis and septic shock: 2012. Crit Care Med 2013;41(2):580–637.

56. Hjortrup PB, Haase N, Bundgaard H, et al. Restricting volumes of resuscitation fluid in adults with septic shock after initial management: the CLASSIC randomised, parallel-group, multicentre feasibility trial. Intensive Care Med 2016; 42(11):1695–705.

57. Damman K, van Deursen VM, Navis G, et al. Increased central venous pressure is associated with impaired renal function and mortality in a broad spectrum of patients with cardiovascular disease. J Am Coll Cardiol 2009;53(7):582–8.

58. Mullens W, Abrahams Z, Francis GS, et al. Importance of venous congestion for worsening of renal function in advanced decompensated heart failure. J Am Coll Cardiol 2009;53(7):589–96.

59. Johnson AEW, Pollard TJ, Shen L, et al. MIMIC-III, a freely accessible critical care database. Sci Data 2016;3:160035.

60. Li DK, Wang XT, Liu DW. Association between elevated central venous pressure and outcomes in critically ill patients. Ann Intensive Care 2017;7(1):83.

61. Parke RL, McGuinness SP, Gilder E, et al. Intravenous fluid use after cardiac surgery: a multicentre, prospective, observational study. Crit Care Resusc 2014; 16(3):164–9.

62. Haase-Fielitz A, Haase M, Bellomo R, et al. Perioperative hemodynamic instability and fluid overload are associated with increasing acute kidney injury severity and worse outcome after cardiac surgery. Blood Purif 2017;43(4): 298–308.

63. Martensson J, Bellomo R. Are all fluids bad for the kidney? Curr Opin Crit Care 2015;21(4):292–301.

64. Singh P, Okusa MD. The role of tubuloglomerular feedback in the pathogenesis of acute kidney injury. Contrib Nephrol 2011;174:12–21.

65. Caironi P, Tognoni G, Masson S, et al. Albumin replacement in patients with severe sepsis or septic shock. N Engl J Med 2014;370(15):1412–21.

66. Charpentier J, Mira J. Efficacy and tolerance of hyperoncotic albumin administration in septic shock patients: the EARSS study [abstract]. Intensive Care Med 2011;37(Supplement 1):S115–0438.

67. Tomita H, Ito U, Tone O, et al. High colloid oncotic therapy for contusional brain edema. Acta Neurochir Suppl (Wien) 1994;60:547–9.

68. Schick MA, Isbary TJ, Schlegel N, et al. The impact of crystalloid and colloid infusion on the kidney in rodent sepsis. Intensive Care Med 2010;36(3):541–8.

69. Wiedermann CJ, Joannidis M. Accumulation of hydroxyethyl starch in human and animal tissues: a systematic review. Intensive Care Med 2014;40(2):160–70.

70. Hammond NE, Taylor C, Finfer S, et al. Patterns of intravenous fluid resuscitation use in adult intensive care patients between 2007 and 2014: an international cross-sectional study. PLoS One 2017;12(5):e0176292.

71. Hammond NE, Taylor C, Saxena M, et al. Resuscitation fluid use in Australian and New Zealand intensive care units between 2007 and 2013. Intensive Care Med 2015;41(9):1611–9.

72. Glassford NJ, French CJ, Bailey M, et al. Changes in intravenous fluid use patterns in Australia and New Zealand: evidence of research translating into practice. Crit Care Resusc 2016;18(2):78–88.

73. Bihari S, Peake SL, Prakash S, et al. Sodium balance, not fluid balance, is associated with respiratory dysfunction in mechanically ventilated patients: a prospective, multicentre study. Crit Care Resusc 2015;17(1):23–8.

74. Bihari S, Peake SL, Seppelt I, et al. Sodium administration in critically ill patients in Australia and New Zealand: a multicentre point prevalence study. Crit Care Resusc 2013;15(4):294–300.

75. Kumar AB, Shi Y, Shotwell MS, et al. Hypernatremia is a significant risk factor for acute kidney injury after subarachnoid hemorrhage: a retrospective analysis. Neurocrit Care 2015;22(2):184–91.

76. Darmon M, Pichon M, Schwebel C, et al. Influence of early dysnatremia correction on survival of critically ill patients. Shock 2014;41(5):394–9.

77. Yunos NM, Bellomo R, Glassford N, et al. Chloride-liberal vs. chloride-restrictive intravenous fluid administration and acute kidney injury: an extended analysis. Intensive Care Med 2015;41(2):257–64.

78. Yunos NM, Bellomo R, Hegarty C, et al. Association between a chloride-liberal vs chloride-restrictive intravenous fluid administration strategy and kidney injury in critically ill adults. JAMA 2012;308(15):1566–72.

79. Yunos NM, Bellomo R, Story D, et al. Bench-to-bedside review: chloride in critical illness. Crit Care 2010;14(4):226.

80. Young P, Bailey M, Beasley R, et al. Effect of a buffered crystalloid solution vs saline on acute kidney injury among patients in the intensive care unit: the SPLIT randomized clinical trial. JAMA 2015;314(16):1701–10.

81. Donner A, Birkett N, Buck C. Randomization by cluster. Sample size requirements and analysis. Am J Epidemiol 1981;114(6):906–14.

82. Connelly LB. Balancing the number and size of sites: an economic approach to the optimal design of cluster samples. Control Clin Trials 2003;24(5):544–59.

83. Semler MW, Wanderer JP, Ehrenfeld JM, et al. Balanced crystalloids versus saline in the intensive care unit. The SALT randomized trial. Am J Respir Crit Care Med 2017;195(10):1362–72.

84. Smith CA, Duby JJ, Utter GH, et al. Cost-minimization analysis of two fluid products for resuscitation of critically injured trauma patients. Am J Health Syst Pharm 2014;71(6):470–5.

85. Semler MW, Self WH, Wang L, et al. Balanced crystalloids versus saline in the intensive care unit: study protocol for a cluster-randomized, multiple-crossover trial. Trials 2017;18(1):129.

86. Hammond NE, Bellomo R, Gallagher M, et al. The Plasma-Lyte 148 v Saline (PLUS) study protocol: a multicentre, randomised controlled trial of the effect of intensive care fluid therapy on mortality. Crit Care Resusc 2017;19(3):239–46.

87. Finfer S, Bellomo R, Boyce N, et al. A comparison of albumin and saline for fluid resuscitation in the intensive care unit. N Engl J Med 2004;350(22):2247–56.

88. Delaney AP, Dan A, McCaffrey J, et al. The role of albumin as a resuscitation fluid for patients with sepsis: a systematic review and meta-analysis. Crit Care Med 2011;39(2):386–91.

89. Myburgh J, Cooper DJ, Finfer S, et al. Saline or albumin for fluid resuscitation in patients with traumatic brain injury. N Engl J Med 2007;357(9):874–84.

90. Finfer S, McEvoy S, Bellomo R, et al. Impact of albumin compared to saline on organ function and mortality of patients with severe sepsis. Intensive Care Med 2011;37(1):86–96.

91. Cooper DJ, Myburgh J, Heritier S, et al. Albumin resuscitation for traumatic brain injury: is intracranial hypertension the cause of increased mortality? J Neurotrauma 2013;30(7):512–8.

92. Maitland K, Akech SO, Russell EC. Mortality after fluid bolus in African children with severe infection: the authors reply. N Engl J Med 2011;365(14):1351–3.

93. Kiguli S, Akech SO, Mtove G, et al. Authors' reply to Southall. BMJ 2014;348: g1619.

94. Kiguli S, Akech SO, Mtove G, et al. WHO guidelines on fluid resuscitation in children: missing the FEAST data. BMJ 2014;348:f7003.

95. Maitland K, Babiker A, Kiguli S, et al. The FEAST trial of fluid bolus in African children with severe infection. Lancet 2012;379(9816):613 [author reply: 613–4].

96. Maitland K, George EC, Evans JA, et al. Exploring mechanisms of excess mortality with early fluid resuscitation: insights from the FEAST trial. BMC Med 2013; 11:68.

97. Maitland K, Kiguli S, Opoka RO, et al. Mortality after fluid bolus in African children with severe infection. N Engl J Med 2011;364(26):2483–95.

98. Glassford NJ, Gelbart B, Bellomo R. Coming full circle: thirty years of paediatric fluid resuscitation. Anaesth Intensive Care 2017;45(3):308–19.

99. Frenette AJ, Bouchard J, Bernier P, et al. Albumin administration is associated with acute kidney injury in cardiac surgery: a propensity score analysis. Crit Care 2014;18(6):602.

100. Mazzocco K, Petitti DB, Fong KT, et al. Surgical team behaviors and patient outcomes. Am J Surg 2009;197(5):678–85.

101. Schortgen F, Girou E, Deye N, et al. The risk associated with hyperoncotic colloids in patients with shock. Intensive Care Med 2008;34(12):2157–68.

102. Bannard-Smith J, Alexander P, Glassford N, et al. Haemodynamic and biochemical responses to fluid bolus therapy with human albumin solution, 4% versus 20%, in critically ill adults. Crit Care Resusc 2015;17(2):122–8.

103. Perner A, Haase N, Guttormsen AB, et al. Hydroxyethyl starch 130/0.42 versus Ringer's acetate in severe sepsis. N Engl J Med 2012;367(2):124–34.

104. Myburgh JA, Finfer S, Bellomo R, et al. Hydroxyethyl starch or saline for fluid resuscitation in intensive care. N Engl J Med 2012;367(20):1901–11.

105. Haase N, Perner A, Hennings LI, et al. Hydroxyethyl starch 130/0.38–0.45 versus crystalloid or albumin in patients with sepsis: systematic review with meta-analysis and trial sequential analysis. BMJ 2013;346:f839.

106. Rochwerg B, Alhazzani W, Gibson A, et al. Fluid type and the use of renal replacement therapy in sepsis: a systematic review and network meta-analysis. Intensive Care Med 2015;41(9):1561–71.

107. Zarychanski R, Abou-Setta AM, Turgeon AF, et al. Association of hydroxyethyl starch administration with mortality and acute kidney injury in critically ill patients requiring volume resuscitation: a systematic review and meta-analysis. JAMA 2013;309(7):678–88.

108. Bellomo R. Starch solutions in Australia: the empire strikes back. Crit Care Resusc 2013;15(4):253–4.

109. Bellomo R, Bion J, Finfer S, et al. Open letter to the executive director of the European Medicines Agency concerning the licensing of hydroxyethyl starch solutions for fluid resuscitation. Acta Anaesthesiol Scand 2014;58(3):365–70.

110. Bellomo R, Bion J, Finfer S, et al. Open letter to the executive director of the European Medicines Agency concerning the licensing of hydroxyethyl starch solutions for fluid resuscitation. Br J Anaesth 2014;112(3):595–600.

111. Patel A, Pieper K, Myburgh JA, et al. Reanalysis of the Crystalloid Versus Hydroxyethyl Starch Trial (CHEST). N Engl J Med 2017;377(3):298–300.

112. Spoelstra-de Man AM, Smorenberg A, Groeneveld AB. Different effects of fluid loading with saline, gelatine, hydroxyethyl starch or albumin solutions on acid-base status in the critically ill. PLoS One 2017;12(4):e0174507.

113. Smorenberg A, Groeneveld AB. Diuretic response to colloid and crystalloid fluid loading in critically ill patients. J Nephrol 2015;28(1):89–95.

114. Pisano A, Landoni G, Bellomo R. The risk of infusing gelatin? Die-hard misconceptions and forgotten (or ignored) truths. Minerva Anestesiol 2016;82(10): 1107–14.

115. Aldecoa C, Kozek-Langenecker S, Rico-Feijoo J. Colloids in surgery: bad drugs, bad protocol, or bad data analysis? Minerva Anestesiol 2014;80(7): 856–7.

116. Food and Drug Administration. List of drug products that have been withdrawn or removed from the market for reasons of safety or effectiveness. 1978. Available at: https://www.fda.gov/ohrms/dockets/98fr/da1008co.pdf. Accessed September 8, 2017.

117. Kozek-Langenecker SA. Fluids and coagulation. Curr Opin Crit Care 2015; 21(4):285–91.

118. Bayer O, Reinhart K, Kohl M, et al. Effects of fluid resuscitation with synthetic colloids or crystalloids alone on shock reversal, fluid balance, and patient outcomes in patients with severe sepsis: a prospective sequential analysis. Crit Care Med 2012;40(9):2543–51.

119. Bayer O, Schwarzkopf D, Doenst T, et al. Perioperative fluid therapy with tetra-starch and gelatin in cardiac surgery–a prospective sequential analysis*. Crit Care Med 2013;41(11):2532–42.

120. Moeller C, Fleischmann C, Thomas-Rueddel D, et al. How safe is gelatin? A systematic review and meta-analysis of gelatin-containing plasma expanders vs crystalloids and albumin. J Crit Care 2016;35:75–83.

121. Perel P, Roberts I, Ker K. Colloids versus crystalloids for fluid resuscitation in critically ill patients. Cochrane Database Syst Rev 2013;(2):CD000567.

Blood Product Administration in the Critical Care and Perioperative Settings

Sofie Louise Rygård, MD[a], Lars Broksø Holst, MD, PhD[a],
Anders Perner, MD, PhD[a,b],*

KEYWORDS

- Critical care • ICU • Perioperative • Plasma • Platelets • Thrombocytes • Anemia
- Red blood cells

KEY POINTS

- Anemia, bleeding, and coagulopathy are frequent in the critical care and perioperative settings.
- Identification of cause is essential for optimal management.
- An imperative restrictive transfusion policy is preferable for all blood products.
- A restrictive hemoglobin level as the threshold for transfusion in all nonbleeding critically ill patients and perioperative patients—with the exception of patients with ongoing myocardial ischemia and patients with traumatic brain injury.
- Only use prophylactic platelet transfusion when total platelet count is below $20 \times 10^9/L$.
- The use of plasma to correct coagulation abnormalities without bleeding is likely of limited benefit.

INTRODUCTION

To enable transfusion of patients, whole blood is collected from healthy volunteers and separated into blood products—plasma, platelets, and red blood cells (RBCs) (**Fig. 1**). The blood is often filtered to reduce the number of immune cells, which may induce adverse effects and transfer DNA from donor to recipient. When transfusing blood products to a patient, weighing the risks and benefits is needed. The final decision should be based on the best available evidence for transfusion of the specific blood product in the specific clinical setting.

Disclosure Statement: The Department of Intensive Care, Rigshospitalet, receives support for research from CSL Behring, Fresenius Kabi, and Ferring Pharmaceuticals.
[a] Department of Intensive Care, Copenhagen University Hospital, Rigshospitalet, Inge Lehmansvej 5, Opg. 3, 3. sal, 4131, Copenhagen Ø 2100, Denmark; [b] Centre for Research in Intensive Care (CRIC), Tagensvej 22, 2200 Copenhagen N, Denmark
* Corresponding author. Department of Intensive Care, Copenhagen University Hospital, Rigshospitalet, Inge Lehmansvej 5, Opg. 3, 3. sal, 4131, Copenhagen Ø 2100, Denmark.
E-mail address: anders.perner@regionh.dk

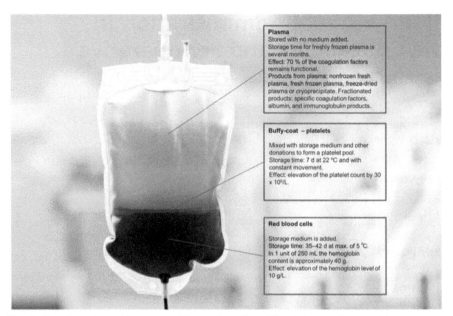

Plasma
Stored with no medium added.
Storage time for freshly frozen plasma is several months.
Effect: 70 % of the coagulation factors remains functional.
Products from plasma: nonfrozen fresh plasma, fresh frozen plasma, freeze-dried plasma or cryoprecipitate. Fractionated products: specific coagulation factors, albumin, and immunoglobulin products.

Buffy-coat – platelets
Mixed with storage medium and other donations to form a platelet pool.
Storage time: 7 d at 22 °C and with constant movement.
Effect: elevation of the platelet count by 30 x 10⁹/L.

Red blood cells
Storage medium is added.
Storage time: 35–42 d at max. of 5 °C.
In 1 unit of 250 mL the hemoglobin content is approximately 40 g.
Effect: elevation of the hemoglobin level of 10 g/L.

Fig. 1. Blood products. (*Courtesy of* Tomas Bertelsen, Blood donors, Denmark.)

Blood products are scarce resources and a significant expenditure for health care systems worldwide. Even though developments in the screening of blood donors and donated blood have resulted in a very low risk of transfusion-transmitted infections, there are still residual risks of adverse reactions when transfusing blood products; the reactions can be mild, moderate, severe, or even life-threatening. Transfusion-related circulatory overload and acute hemolytic transfusion reactions are the main causes of transfusion-related deaths,[1] and a majority of these events are due to human errors and are preventable when correct evaluation of the prescription and checking is performed before transfusion. The risk of serious transfusion-related harm is approximately 1 in 15,000 transfusion events and the risk of death related to transfusion events is estimated at 1 in 100,000.[1]

During storage, the RBC changes shape and function, and substances are leaked from the cell into the storage medium—changes that combined are called the "storage lesion."[2] In vitro studies have shown the changes to compromise the functionality of the RBC,[3] and several observational studies and randomized clinical trials (RCTs) have investigated the in vivo effect of storage on clinical outcomes.

The donation of blood by millions of healthy volunteers daily is also associated with complications. Up to one-third of donors may experience adverse effects, for example, iron deficiency, vasovagal reactions, and local symptoms, although the majority is of mild character.[4]

Regarding blood donors putting themselves at risk, the expensive and limited resource of blood products, and the known and hidden adverse effects of transfusion, an imperative non-overtransfusion policy is preferable for all blood products.

The critical care and perioperative settings are high consumers of blood products, with multiple units and different products often given to an individual patient. Packed RBCs are the most frequent product used in ICUs and in the perioperative setting[5]; the use of blood products in these settings is described. Trauma and massive transfusion, discussed in detail in a recent publication by Chang and Holcomb,[6] are not discussed in this article.

OVERVIEW OF THE CRITICAL CARE SETTING

The RBC transfusion rate is approximately 37% to 44% in the general ICU population[7,8] and higher in some subgroups of patients (eg, patients with sepsis[9]). The most common indications for RBC transfusion are anemia and bleeding. The causes of anemia are multifactorial (**Fig. 2**). Different approaches to correct anemia have been investigated, including the use of intravenous (IV) iron[10,11] and erythropoietin-stimulating agents,[12–14] but at present there are no firm evidence for benefit of these approaches.[15–17] Currently, transfusion with RBC units is the only way to urgently correct anemia.

Coagulopathy is another common condition encountered in the ICU, where coagulation factors, platelets, or coagulation pathways are dysfunctional, resulting in various clinical consequences (see Table 1).[19] In a large UK cohort study, the prevalence of severe thrombocytopenia (platelets $<50 \times 10^9$/L) was 12% during ICU admission.[18] The causes may relate to mechanical or immunologic processes, drug side effects, and/or diseases like disseminated intravascular coagulation, liver failure, cancer, and hematological diseases.[19] In the UK cohort, 9% of all patients received a median of 2 platelet transfusions, and more than half of the transfusions were given on days with no clinically significant bleeding,[18] indicating frequent use of prophylactic platelet transfusion.

The use of plasma in the ICU is primarily due to bleeding or coagulopathy; overall, approximately 13% of ICU patients receive a plasma transfusion.[20] Among patients with septic shock, an even higher transfusion rate of 57% has been reported, with a median of 6 units of plasma per patient.[21] Other studies have indicated a high number of inappropriate transfusions,[22,23] but this area lacks data from high-quality studies.[24]

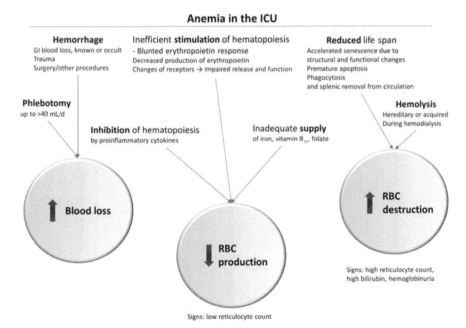

Fig. 2. Anemia in the ICU. GI, gastrointestinal.

OVERVIEW OF THE PERIOPERATIVE SETTING

Preoperative anemia may be present in up to one-third of surgical patients, with a higher rate in, for example, cardiac surgery,[25] and after surgery even more patients are anemic. Even mild degrees of anemia are associated with worse patient outcome,[26,27] but in elective surgery, there is the possibility of preoperative optimization of the hemoglobin (Hb) level, and this may improve outcomes.[28]

Patient blood management (PBM) is a multidisciplinary clinical approach aiming to improve patient outcome by putting patients at the center of transfusion management to give the right products to the right patients at the right time.[29,30] PBM builds in general on 3 pillars: optimizing a patient's blood volume and red cell mass, minimizing the loss of blood, and optimizing a patient's tolerance of anemia (**Fig. 3**).

Preoperative anemia has been strongly correlated with perioperative RBC transfusion,[25] but the transfusion rate differs considerably between different degrees of anemia and different centers.[27,28,31] A recent European survey of the clinical practice in perioperative PBM reported that more than half of physicians used a level of 70 g/L Hb to 90 g/L Hb as transfusion threshold, and approximately one-third used a level of more than 90 g/L.[32]

Bleeding during surgery can be anticipated and seen as a consequence of complications, and the amount of blood loss varies between surgical specialties and procedures. In another recent European survey of patients receiving RBC transfusions, a mean blood loss during surgery of 1392 mL was observed, and almost half of the patients also received either plasma or platelet transfusions.[33]

MANAGEMENT IN CRITICAL ILLNESS

There are several strategies to administrating blood products in a restrictive manner in an ICU. First, prevention of the need for a blood product is essential. Second, when there is a need, the cause should be identified and sought to be corrected, if possible.

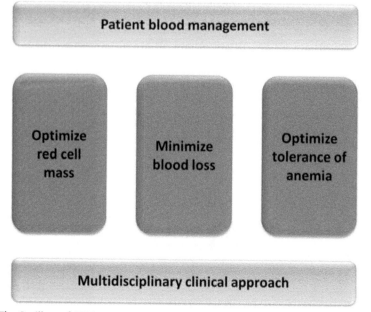

Fig. 3. The 3 pillars of PBM.

Third, when administrating blood products, clinicians should be guided by the available high-quality evidence regarding the blood product and patient category.

Anemia

Anemia or worsening of anemia can be prevented by minimizing the volume of blood drawn daily from patients in the ICU. Critical evaluation of the need for routine laboratory test, blood cultures, and point-of-care testing alongside the use of pediatric tubes and blood-saving devices can reduce the volume of blood taken from ICU patients.[34]

Identification of the causes of anemia can be complex in the critical care setting,[35] but an important issue to investigate is the presence of iron deficiency with a potential of correcting by administrating oral or IV iron.[36] In the IRONMAN (Intravenous Iron or Placebo for Anaemia in Intensive Care) trial, the administration of IV iron did not decrease the number of RBC units transfused, but a significant increase in Hb level at hospital discharge was observed in the intervention versus the placebo group.[11] The diagnosis of true iron deficiency in the ICU is difficult; this area has been discussed in detail in a previous review by Prakash.[35]

The use of erythropoietin-stimulating agents is not recommended in critically ill patients, due to lack of efficacy and unclear risk of harm.[15]

Red Blood Cell Administration

The indications for RBC transfusions in the general ICU population are acute bleeding with hemodynamically instability or anemia with an Hb level of less than 70 g/L.[37–39] Evidence on safety using a restrictive transfusion strategy in the ICU is primarily based on the results from 2 large RCTs.[40] The TRICC (Transfusion Requirements In Critical Care) trial, conducted in a general, Canadian ICU population, showed effectiveness and safety of using a restrictive transfusion strategy (Hb level 70 g/L) and even signs of superiority in some subgroups of patients (younger and less critically ill) than a liberal transfusion strategy (90 g/L).[37] The TRISS (Transfusion Requirements in Septic Shock) trial, 15 years later used the same threshold levels as for transfusion in patients with septic shock.[39] The results showed that in a patient population with severe critical illness, the restrictive transfusion strategy led to fewer patients transfused and fewer RBC units transfused, with outcomes similar to those of patients treated with the more liberal transfusion strategy.[39]

The evidence for the optimal use of RBC transfusion in ICU patients with acute cardiovascular disease or with chronic cardiovascular disease (CVD) is sparse.[41] These patient populations were only represented in small subgroups in the trials discussed previously, and non-ICU trials and a meta-analysis have suggested a benefit of a more liberal strategy in CVD patients regarding morbidity and the development of new ischemic events.[42–44] Until firm evidence on safety is present, patients with ongoing acute coronary syndrome may be transfused more liberally aiming for a higher Hb level.

Evidence is also lacking on how to manage patients with traumatic brain injury (TBI). Two trials have investigated the optimal Hb level for transfusion in this patient population, Zygun and colleagues[45] in 2009 and Robertson and colleagues[46] in 2014. In the first trial, 30 patients with severe TBI were transfused at 3 different Hb levels (80 g/L, 90 g/L, and 100 g/L) to evaluate the effect on brain tissue oxygenation.[45] The results showed that RBC transfusion at the higher levels was associated with higher brain tissue oxygenation, but the trial was not powered to assess effects on any patient-important outcome measures.[45] The second trial had a factorial design where 200 patients with closed head injury were treated with erythropoietin or placebo and with RBC transfusion at an Hb level of 70 g/L or 100 g/L.[46] The results showed no beneficial effect of either erythropoietin nor liberal transfusion.[46] Because the evidence is sparse, further trials with low risk of bias are needed to determine the optimal Hb threshold for transfusion in patients with TBI.

For both acute coronary syndrome and TBI, an Hb level of 80 g/L for transfusion may be used until the safety of a more restrictive threshold is shown.

Patients with chronic anemia receiving frequent RBC transfusions, such as patients with cancer, hematological malignancies, or chronic renal disease, should be evaluated individually, and a consensus stated on the Hb level to trigger transfusion. A restrictive transfusion strategy seems safe in patients with cancer and hematological diseases,[47] although there is limited high-quality evidence on this area.[48,49]

Regarding the effect of RBC storage time on patient-important outcomes, there is now high-quality evidence from 2 large RCTs conducted in the ICU, the ABLE (Age of Blood Evaluation) trial and the TRANSFUSE (Standard Issue Transfusion Versus Fresher Red Blood Cell Use in Intensive Care) trial.[50,51] Both showed no beneficial effect of fresher blood; rather, the point estimates for the risk of death favored older blood in both trials.[50,51] Hence, the debate of the harmful effect of older versus fresher blood seems closed, and the practice of using the oldest available RBC unit first seems safe.

To further minimize the blood product use, all nonbleeding patients should be treated with single-unit transfusions followed by assessment of patient clinical status and a renewed test of the Hb level.

The Use of Plasma and Platelets

Patients should be evaluated for the causes of coagulopathies and followed closely, especially for their risk of bleeding. But neither plasma nor platelets should be administered routinely to correct coagulopathies.

The current use of plasma, prophylactic or therapeutic, is not supported by any solid evidence regarding safety or effect.[24,52,53] There are known risks of plasma transfusions (transfusion-related acute lung injury and severe allergic reactions), and until further knowledge is established, the authors recommend a restrictive use of plasma. Viscoelastic hemostatic assays (VHAs) together with standard laboratory parameters may be used to guide plasma transfusions in bleeding patients.[54]

Platelet use is also either prophylactic or therapeutic—by preventing or treating bleeding—and in general the evidence for the optimal platelet level as trigger for transfusion of platelets is of low quality or very low quality.[55] The platelet count and the platelet function can both or separately be affected, and the causes should be investigated. To investigate the function of the platelets, the authors recommend the use of VHA when a platelet transfusion is considered, and, in line with different national guidelines, the authors recommend not to use prophylactic platelet transfusion to reduce bleeding risk in nonbleeding patients until the platelet count is less than $20 \times 10^9/L$.[55,56]

PERIOPERATIVE MANAGEMENT

Management of blood product administration before, during, and after surgery should be guided by the principles of PBM.

Preoperative Optimization

Anemia

Anemia should be identified, evaluated, and managed 3 weeks to 8 weeks prior to surgery to optimize patients.[57] A thorough overview of the diagnosis and management of iron deficiency anemia is available,[58] and a guideline to the preoperatively management has been presented by the National Blood Authority of Australia (**Fig. 4**).[59] In cases of more urgent surgical procedures, where time to correct anemia is limited, the use of IV

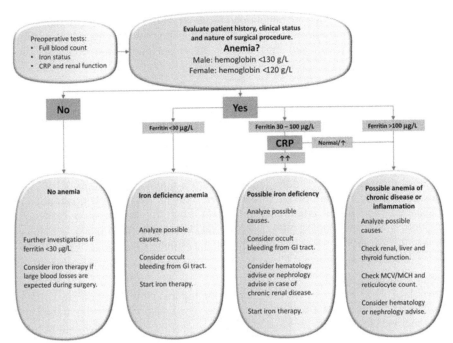

Fig. 4. The preoperative assessment and handling of anemia. CRP, C-reactive protein; GI, gastrointestinal; MCH, mean corpuscular Hb; MCV, mean corpuscular volume. (*Adapted from* National Blood Authority. Patient blood management guidelines: module 2 perioperative. 2012. Available at: www.nba.gov.au. Accessed September 1, 2017.)

iron may be considered. In a recent RCT, adult patients with iron deficiency anemia scheduled for abdominal surgery were randomized to either usual care or substitution with IV iron perioperatively.[60] The use of IV iron resulted in a lower transfusion rate and higher Hb level 4 weeks postsurgery. They observed no effects on 30-day mortality or quality of life, but the trial was ended prematurely due to an interim analysis, when only approximately 25% of the intended number of patients were included.[60] IV iron can be considered when oral iron is contradicted, not tolerated, or not effective and in case surgery cannot be postponed.

Risk of bleeding
The risks of bleeding should be identified before surgery, including those for the specific surgical procedure, those due to coagulations disorders or anticoagulant drug therapy, those due to other comorbidities, and importantly those related to any history of bleeding, family bleeding history, or medications; a full list should be used for the risk assessment.[57]

One approach to handle the risk of expected bleeding and need for an RBC transfusion is the use of a patient's own blood reserve by autologous blood donations presurgery, known as isovolemic hemodilution, but the efficacy of this approach is not well documented, and it has even been shown to increase the risk of being transfused and, therefore, is not recommended.[61–63]

In cases of oral anticoagulant therapy, consideration of bridging with heparin could be commenced in patients with high risk of thromboembolism, but the evidence in this field is less clear.[64] The recent BRIDGE (Bridging Anticoagulation in Patients who Require Temporary Interruption of Warfarin Therapy for an Elective Invasive Procedure or Surgery) trial indicated noninferiority regarding arterial thromboembolism or bleeding of no-bridging versus bridging with low-molecular-weight heparin in patients with atrial fibrillation who had their warfarin treatment interrupted during elective surgery.[65]

Intraoperative Management

During surgery, the clinical status of a patient together with the Hb level can be used as trigger for RBC transfusion. There are conflicting results from RCTs in the perioperative setting investigating the effectiveness and safety of a restrictive versus a liberal transfusion strategy.[40,66] Most of the trials in the perioperative setting included patients postoperatively, but there is some consensus for a restrictive Hb threshold of 70 g/L during surgery, with a target of 70 g/L to 90 g/L with active bleeding.[57,67] The optimal threshold for patients with CVD is again not well established, and these patients may benefit from transfusion at a higher Hb threshold.[43] A large ongoing study will add valuable evidence to guide transfusion perioperatively (Transfusion Requirements in Cardiac Surgery [TRICS] III trial, NCT02042898).

Bleeding during surgery

Minimizing blood loss can be effectuated by reducing the intraoperative risk of bleeding and by reuse of a patient's own blood. The antifibrinolytic drug, tranexamic acid, seems safe to use in all surgical patients, including trauma patients and those undergoing cardiac surgery,[68,69] to reduce rate of bleeding and reduci the need for blood product transfusion.[70] The safety and effectiveness of tranexamic acid among patients with TBI and gastrointestinal bleeding are still under investigation in large RCTs.[71,72]

In a subgroup of critically ill surgical patients, Villanueva and colleagues[67] showed that patients with upper gastrointestinal bleeding randomized to a restrictive (70 g/L) Hb threshold for transfusion had lower 45-day mortality versus those randomized to a liberal (90 g/L) threshold.

Perioperative blood loss can be reused by cell salvage through collection, filtration, and reinfusion of the blood into a patient. This procedure has shown efficacy regarding the minimization of blood product transfusions without adversely affecting patient outcome, but evidence has low quality.[73]

Intraoperative bleeding is either due to lack of surgical hemostasis or a nonsurgical bleeding due to coagulopathies and a patient's inability to form clots. In the latter situation, goal-directed hemostatic treatment may be guided by VHA and traditional laboratory parameters.[74]

Postoperative Management

Postoperative bleeding may occur, and the use of VHA may be continued to follow the coagulation status. Importantly, patients in general shift from a state of relative anticoagulation into a hyperinflammatory prothrombotic phase, and prophylactic anticoagulant treatment should be reinstituted or commenced.

The FOCUS (Transfusion Trigger Trial for Functional Outcomes in Cardiovascular Patients Undergoing Surgical Hip Fracture Repair) trial randomized nonbleeding elderly patients with mild to severe CVD to an Hb threshold of 80 g/L or 100 g/L for transfusion after total hip replacement surgery.[75] The primary outcome of 60-day mortality and the inability to walk independently did not differ between the groups; neither did long-term mortality or causes of death.[76] In general, postoperative transfusion strategies should be restrictive.

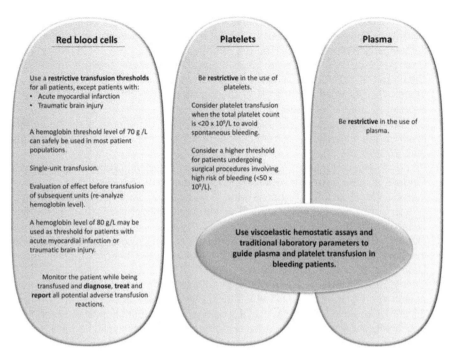

Fig. 5. Summary of recommendations.

PERSPECTIVE

There are still several areas in the use of blood products that need further investigation. With the high incidence of anemia, coagulopathy, and bleeding and the large consumption of blood products in the critical care and the perioperative settings, there is a great opportunity to evaluate the indications and optimal thresholds for transfusion of different blood products.

The important recommendation of this review is to consider the risks and benefits for specific blood products for specific patients in specific clinical settings (**Fig. 5**). Optimize patient status by treating anemia and preventing the need for RBC transfusion. Consider other options for correction of anemia and coagulation disorders—maybe a wait-and-see approach is of more benefit for patients than over-treating with blood products—with regards to donors, society, and patients.

REFERENCES

1. Bolton-Maggs PHB, Poles D, et al, editors, on behalf of the Serious Hazards of Transfusion (SHOT) Steering Group. The 2015 Annual SHOT report (2016). 2016. Available at: http://www.shotuk.org. Accessed September 1, 2017.
2. Wolfe LC. The membrane and the lesions of storage in preserved red cells. Transfusion 1985;25(3):185–203.
3. Berezina TL, Zaets SB, Morgan C, et al. Influence of storage on red blood cell rheological properties. J Surg Res 2002;102:6–12.
4. Amrein K, Valentin A, Lanzer G, et al. Blood reviews adverse events and safety issues in blood donation — a comprehensive review. Blood Rev 2012;26:33–42.

5. Department of health and human services. The 2011 National Blood Collection and Utilization Survey Report. 2011. Available at: https://www.aabb.org/research/hemovigilance/bloods. Accessed September 1, 2017.

6. Chang R, Holcomb JB. Optimal fluid therapy for traumatic hemorrhagic shock. Crit Care Clin 2017;33(1):15–36.

7. Vincent JL, Baron J-F, Reinhart K, et al. Anemia and blood transfusion in critically ill patients. JAMA 2002;288(12):1499–507.

8. Corwin HL, Gettinger A, Pearl RG, et al. The CRIT study: anemia and blood transfusion in the critically ill - current clinical practice in the United States. Crit Care Med 2004;32:39–52.

9. Perner A, Haase N, Guttormsen AB, et al. Hydroxyethyl starch 130/0.42 versus Ringer's acetate in severe sepsis. N Engl J Med 2012;367(2):82–3.

10. Pieracci FM, Stovall RT, Jaouen B, et al. A multicenter, randomized clinical trial of IV iron supplementation for anemia of traumatic critical illness. Crit Care Med 2014;42(6):1–10.

11. Litton E, Baker S, Erber WN, et al. Intravenous iron or placebo for anaemia in intensive care: the IRONMAN multicentre randomized blinded trial. Intensive Care Med 2016;42(11):1715–22.

12. Corwin HL, Gettinger A, Pearl RG, et al. Efficacy of recombinant human erythropoietin in critically ill patients. JAMA 2002;288(22):2827–35.

13. Silver M, Corwin MJ, Bazan A, et al. Efficacy of recombinant human erythropoietin in critically ill patients admitted to a long-term acute care facility: a randomized, double-blind, placebo-controlled trial. Crit Care Med 2006;34(9):2310–6.

14. Corwin HL, Gettinger A, Fabian T, et al. Efficacy and safety of epoetin alfa in critically ill patients. N Engl J Med 2007;357(10):965–76.

15. Zarychanski R, Turgeon AF, McIntyre LA, et al. Erythropoietin-receptor agonists in critically ill patients: a meta-analysis of randomized controlled trials. Can Med Assoc J 2007;177(7):725–34.

16. Zhao C, Lin Z, Luo Q, et al. Efficacy and safety of erythropoietin to prevent acute kidney injury in patients with critical illness or perioperative care: a systematic review and meta-analysis of randomized controlled trials. J Cardiovasc Pharmacol 2015; 65(6):593–600.

17. Shah A, Roy NB, McKechnie S, et al. Iron supplementation to treat anaemia in adult critical care patients: a systematic review and meta-analysis. Crit Care 2016;20(1):306.

18. Stanworth SJ, Walsh TS, Prescott RJ, et al. Thrombocytopenia and platelet transfusion in UK critical care: a multicenter observational study. Transfusion 2013;53:1050–8.

19. Hunt BJ. Bleeding and coagulopathies in critical care. N Engl J Med 2014;370:847–59.

20. Stanworth SJ, Walsh TS, Prescott RJ, et al. A national study of plasma use in critical care: clinical indications, dose and effect on prothrombin time. Crit Care 2011;15(2):R108.

21. Reiter N, Wesche N, Perner A. The majority of patients in septic shock are transfused with fresh-frozen plasma. Dan Med J 2013;60(4):4–7.

22. Dara S, Rana R, Afessa B, et al. Fresh frozen plasma transfusion in critically ill medical patients with coagulopathy. Crit Care Med 2005;33(11):2667–71.

23. Tinmouth A, Thompson T, Arnold DM, et al. Utilization of frozen plasma in Ontario: a provincewide audit reveals a high rate of inappropriate transfusions. Transfusion 2013;53:2222–9.

24. Karam O, Tucci M, Combescure C, et al. Plasma transfusion strategies for critically ill patients (review). Cochrane Database Syst Rev 2013;(12):CD010654.

25. Shander A, Knight K, Thurer R, et al. Prevalence and outcomes of anemia in surgery: a systematic review of the literature. Am J Med 2004;116(7A):58s–69s.

26. Fowler AJ, Ahmad T, Phull MK, et al. Meta-analysis of the association between pre-operative anaemia and mortality after surgery. Br J Surg 2015;102(11):1314–24.

27. Musallam KM, Tamim HM, Richards T, et al. Preoperative anaemia and postoperative outcomes in non-cardiac surgery: a retrospective cohort study. Lancet 2017;378(9800):1396–407.

28. Kotze A, Carter L, Scally A. Effect of a patient blood management programme on preoperative anaemia, transfusion rate, and outcome after primary hip or knee arthroplasty: a quality improvement cycle. Br J Anaesth 2012;108(6):943–52.

29. Goodnough LT, Shander A, Spence R. Bloodless medicine: clinical care without allogeneic blood transfusion. Transfusion 2003;43(5):668–76.

30. Goodnough LT, Shander A. Patient blood management. Anesthesiology 2012; 116(6):1367–76.

31. Norgaard A, De Lichtenberg TH, Nielsen J, et al. Monitoring compliance with transfusion guidelines in hospital departments by electronic data capture. Blood Transfus 2014;12(4):509–19.

32. Baron DM, Metnitz PGH, Fellinger T, et al. Evaluation of clinical practice in perioperative patient blood management. Br J Anaesth 2016;117(5):610–6.

33. Meier J, Filipescu D, Pitarch JL, et al. Intraoperative transfusion practices in Europe. Br J Anaesth 2016;116(2):255–61.

34. Fischer DP, Zacharowski KD, Meybohm P. Savoring every drop – vampire or mosquito? Crit Care 2014;18(306):1–6.

35. Prakash D. Anemia in the ICU: anemia of chronic disease versus anemia of acute illness. Crit Care Clin 2012;28(3):333–43.

36. Heming N, Montravers P, Lasocki S. Iron deficiency in critically ill patients: highlighting the role of hepcidin. Crit Care 2011;15(2):210.

37. Hébert PC, Wells G, Blajchman M, et al. A multicenter, randomized, controlled clinical trial of transfusion requirements in critical care. N Engl J Med 1999; 340(6):409–17.

38. Walsh TS, Boyd JA, Watson D, et al, RELIEVE Investigators. Restrictive versus liberal transfusion strategies for older mechanically ventilated critically ill patients: a randomized pilot trial. Crit Care Med 2013;41(10):2354–63.

39. Holst LB, Haase N, Wetterslev J, et al. Lower versus higher hemoglobin threshold for transfusion in septic shock. N Engl J Med 2014;371(15):1381–91.

40. Holst LB, Petersen MW, Haase N, et al. Restrictive versus liberal transfusion strategy for red blood cell transfusion: systematic review of randomised trials with meta-analysis and trial sequential analysis. BMJ 2015;350:h1354.

41. Docherty AB, Walsh TS. Anemia and blood transfusion in the critically ill patient with cardiovascular disease. Crit Care 2017;21(1):61.

42. Carson JL, Brooks M, Abbott J, et al. Liberal versus restrictive transfusion thresholds for patients with symptomatic coronary artery disease. Am Heart J 2013; 165(6):964–71.

43. Murphy GJ, Pike K, Rogers CA, et al. Liberal or restrictive transfusion after cardiac surgery. N Engl J Med 2015;372(11):997–1008.

44. Docherty AB, O'Donnell R, Brunskill S, et al. Effect of restrictive versus liberal transfusion strategies on outcomes in patients with cardiovascular disease in a non-cardiac surgery setting: systematic review and meta-analysis. BMJ 2016; 352:i1351.

45. Zygun DA, Nortje J, Hutchinson PJ, et al. The effect of red blood cell transfusion on cerebral oxygenation and metabolism after severe traumatic brain injury. Crit Care Med 2009;37(3):1074–8.

46. Robertson C, Hannay J, Yamal J, et al. Effect of erythropoietin administration and after traumatic brain injury: a randomized clinical trial. JAMA 2014;312(1): 36–47.

47. Hoeks MPA, Kranenburg FJ, Middelburg RA, et al. Impact of red blood cell transfusion strategies in haemato-oncological patients: a systematic review and meta-analysis. Br J Haematol 2017;178(1):137–51.

48. Prescott LS, Taylor JS, Lopez-Olivo MA, et al. How low should we go: a systematic review and meta-analysis of the impact of restrictive red blood cell transfusion strategies in oncology. Cancer Treat Rev 2016;46:1–8.

49. Roubinian N, Carson JL. Red blood cell transfusion strategies in adult and pediatric patients with malignancy. Hematol Oncol Clin North Am 2016;30(3):529–40.

50. Lacroix J, Hebert PC, Fergusson DA, et al. Age of transfused blood in critically ill adults. N Engl J Med 2015;372(15):1410–8.

51. Cooper DJ, McQuilten ZK, Nichol A, et al. Age of red cells for transfusion and outcomes in critically ill adults. N Engl J Med 2017;377(19):1858–67.

52. Yang L, Stanworth S, Hopewell S, et al. Is fresh-frozen plasma clinically effective? An update of a systematic review of randomized controlled trials. Transfusion 2012;52(8):1673–86.

53. Hall D, Estcourt L, Doree C, et al. Plasma transfusions prior to insertion of central lines for people with abnormal coagulation (Review). Cochrane Database Syst Rev 2016;(9):CD011756.

54. Durila M, Lukáš P, Astraverkhava M, et al. Tracheostomy in intensive care unit patients can be performed without bleeding complications in case of normal thromboelastometry results (EXTEM CT) despite increased PT-INR: a prospective pilot study. BMC Anesthesiol 2015;15(1):89.

55. Kaufman RM, Djulbegovic B, Gernsheimer T, et al. Platelet transfusion: a clinical practice guideline from the AABB. Ann Intern Med 2015;162:205–13.

56. National Blood Authority. Patient blood management guidelines: module 4-critical care. 2012;1–16. Available at: www.nba.gov.au. Accessed September 1, 2017.

57. Kozek-Langenecker SA, Ahmed AB, Afshari A, et al. Management of severe perioperative bleeding: guidelines from the European Society of Anaesthesiology First update 2016. Eur J Anaesthesiol 2017;34:332–95.

58. Pasricha S-RS, Flecknoe-Brown SC, Allen KJ, et al. Diagnosis and management of iron deficiency anaemia: a clinical update. Med J Aust 2010;193(9):525–32.

59. National Blood Authority. Patient blood management guidelines: module 2 perioperative. 2012. Available at: www.nba.gov.au. Accessed September 1, 2017.

60. Froessler B, Palm P, Weber I, et al. The important role for intravenous iron in perioperative patient blood management in major abdominal surgery. Ann Surg 2016;264(1):41–6.

61. Henry DA, Carless PA, Moxey AJ, et al. Pre-operative autologous donation for minimising perioperative allogeneic blood transfusion. Cochrane Database Syst Rev 2001;(4):CD003602.

62. Bouchard D, Marcheix B, Al-Shamary S, et al. Preoperative autologous blood donation reduces the need for allogeneic blood products: a prospective randomized study. Can J Surg 2008;51(6):422–7.

63. Jakovina Blazekovic S, Bicanic G, Hrabac P, et al. Pre-operative autologous blood donation versus no blood donation in total knee arthroplasty: a prospective randomised trial. Int Orthop 2014;38(2):341–6.

64. Daniels PR. Peri-procedural management of patients taking oral anticoagulants. BMJ 2015;351:h2391.

65. Douketis JD, Spyropoulos AC, Kaatz S, et al. Perioperative bridging anticoagulation in patients with atrial fibrillation. N Engl J Med 2015;373(9):823–33.
66. Fominskiy E, Putzu A, Monaco F, et al. Liberal transfusion strategy improves survival in perioperative but not in critically ill patients. A meta-analysis of randomised trials. Br J Anaesth 2015;115(4):511–9.
67. Villanueva C, Colomo A, Bosch A, et al. Transfusion strategies for acute upper gastrointestinal bleeding. N Engl J Med 2013;368:11–21.
68. Roberts I, Shakur H, Coats T, et al. The CRASH-2 trial: a randomised controlled trial and economic evaluation of the effects of tranexamic acid on death, vascular occlusive events and transfusion requirement in bleeding trauma patients. Health Technol Assess 2013;17(10):1–80.
69. Myles PS, Smith JA, Forbes A, et al. Tranexamic acid in patients undergoing coronary-artery surgery. N Engl J Med 2017;376(2):136–48.
70. Henry DA, Carless PA, Moxey AJ, et al. Anti-fibrinolytic use for minimising perioperative allogeneic blood transfusion (Review) Anti-fibrinolytic use for minimising perioperative allogeneic blood transfusion. Cochrane Database Syst Rev 2011;(1):CD001886.
71. Dewan Y, Komolafe EO, Mejía-Mantilla JH, et al. CRASH-3-tranexamic acid for the treatment of significant traumatic brain injury: study protocol for an international randomized, double-blind, placebo-controlled trial. Trials 2012;13(1):87.
72. Roberts I, Coats T, Edwards P, et al. HALT-IT- tranexamic acid for the treatment of gastrointestinal bleeding: study protocol for a randomised controlled trial. Trials 2014;15(1):450.
73. Carless PA, Henry DA, Moxey AJ, et al. Cell salvage for minimising perioperative allogeneic blood transfusion. Cochrane Database Syst Rev 2010;(3):CD001888.
74. Wikkelsø A, Wetterslev J, Møller A, et al. Thromboelastography (TEG) or thromboelastometry (ROTEM) to monitor haemostatic treatment versus usual care in adults or children with bleeding. Cochrane Database Syst Rev 2016;(8):CD007871.
75. Carson JL, Terrin ML, Noveck H, et al. Liberal or restrictive transfusion in high-risk patients after hip surgery. N Engl J Med 2011;365(26):2453–62.
76. Carson JL, Sieber F, Cook DR, et al. Liberal versus restrictive blood transfusion strategy: 3-year survival and cause of death results from the FOCUS randomised controlled trial. Lancet 2015;385:1183–9.

Moving?

Make sure your subscription moves with you!

To notify us of your new address, find your **Clinics Account Number** (located on your mailing label above your name), and contact customer service at:

Email: journalscustomerservice-usa@elsevier.com

800-654-2452 (subscribers in the U.S. & Canada)
314-447-8871 (subscribers outside of the U.S. & Canada)

Fax number: 314-447-8029

Elsevier Health Sciences Division
Subscription Customer Service
3251 Riverport Lane
Maryland Heights, MO 63043

*To ensure uninterrupted delivery of your subscription, please notify us at least 4 weeks in advance of move.

Printed and bound by CPI Group (UK) Ltd, Croydon, CR0 4YY

03/10/2024

01040391-0011